W9-AOR-072

# FISHBEIN'S *Illustrated*

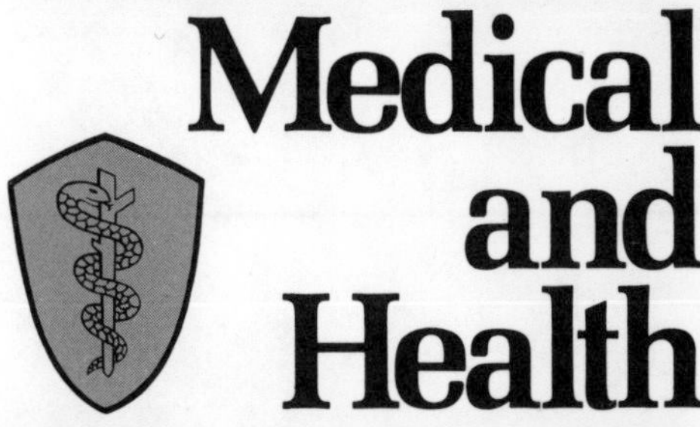


# Encyclopedia

# Fishbein's

# *Illustrated* Medical

**INTERNATIONAL**

*Unified*

**EDITION**

CONTAINS ALL THE A TO Z ENCYCLOPEDIC ENTRIES OF THE HOME LIBRARY EDITION PLUS CONSULTING DISCUSSIONS ON THE MAJOR MEDICAL SPECIALTIES AND MEDICAL SCIENCE PROFILES FROM THE MIND ALIVE ENCYCLOPEDIA

# and Health Encyclopedia

AN AUTHORITATIVE MEDICAL AND HEALTH GUIDE FOR THE FAMILY
PUBLISHED IN COOPERATION WITH A BOARD OF
PHYSICIANS, SURGEONS AND MEDICAL CONSULTANTS

**VOLUME**

**1**

**ABASIA**
**AGUE**

**H. S. STUTTMAN INC.**, Publishers • **WESTPORT, CONNECTICUT 06889**

ISBN 0-87475-200-0

Library of Congress Catalog Card No. 80-52999



Anatomical line illustrations, with the exception of MEDIGRAPH CHARTS, were produced by Mr. Leonard Dank, of Medical Illustration Studio, St. Luke's Hospital.

Many photographs not otherwise credited were produced by Three Lions, Inc. and Susan Faludi.

Text and illustrations making up the MEDICAL SCIENCE PROFILES were first published by MARSHALL CAVENDISH LIMITED in the series *Mind Alive* and are used herein with the permission of the publishers.

PRINTED IN THE UNITED STATES OF AMERICA
4P (0281) 45M-205

# INTRODUCTION

THIS LATEST EDITION of *Fishbein's Illustrated Medical and Health Encyclopedia* is based on the unified concept originated by Dr. Morris Fishbein. A glance at the Table of Contents of this "unified" edition will demonstrate why this concept is the editorial equivalent of a modern consultation and diagnostic clinic.

The greatest fears of humankind are the fears of pain, disease and death. We fear the things that we do not understand much more than we fear the things of which we have full knowledge. With public awareness of the expansion of medical knowledge, and awareness within the medical profession of a "patient's right to know," the "unified" concept embodied in this edition of *Fishbein's Illustrated Medical and Health Encyclopedia* recognizes this most significant right of a patient.

Physiologists understand the importance of feedback to proper function of the human body. So too, reader feedback was equally as important in dictating the format and content of this new unified edition of *Fishbein's Illustrated Medical and Health Encyclopedia.* An awareness of this "reader feedback" guided the writers, researchers, medical consultants and illustrators in their efforts to overcome areas of uncertainty, eliminate confusion and fill in gaps of knowledge. As patients become more and more aware of the expansion of medical knowledge, the questions they raise become more penetrating.

If we were to characterize the major difference of this new unified edition of *Fishbein's Illustrated Medical and Health Encyclopedia* to previous editions, it would be the striking trend toward conveying information in depth. This is evident in each of the 22 volumes as you can readily observe by consulting the Table of Contents. You will understand why mere definitions and basic information by themselves no longer suffice. Now a patient who has penetrating questions is able to obtain comprehensive, authoritative and outspoken answers in the unified editorial and pictorial features included in this edition.

Now, within the framework of an A through Z sequence of authoritative basic information, on major medical conditions from ABASIA to ZYME, the reader can expand his or her understanding and acquire greater depth of medical knowledge. The unified features represent the advice, guidance, research and viewpoints of leading specialists in medicine and surgery.

One of the goals in the preparation of this "unified" edition is to demonstrate that the expanson of medical knowledge is an ongoing phenomenon. It is especially exciting and also comforting to see how medical research holds forth hope for the elimination of so much human suffering. Hence, this new work has included reports on the most significant research in each major medical area. These Research Reports are distributed under the most logical entry in the alphabetic sequence. They are also cross indexed following those entries that have some relationship to the research discussed in the Report. By their very nature, they must be more technical than the main body of encyclopedic entries. They are intended to be reports on research and therefore some of the information may still be in the testing stage rather than for immediate application. They are included for the purpose of giving hints as to the possibilities of such new developments.

An outstandng feature of this new work is the great emphasis placed upon graphics. No effort has been spared to employ every illustrative technique that will tend to make scientific medical information understandable and meaningful to the lay reader. To attain this end, we commissioned a highly qualified medically trained illustrator to create an entire collection of anatomically accurate medical illustrations. These were judiciously used to supplement each pertinent entry where an understanding of the anatomy, systemic function or organ involved would enable the reader to better understand the subject matter. In addition to these anatomical illustrations, each major article that fully describes a specific medical condition is supplemented by a full page Medigraph Chart. This graphic teaching device explains the sequence of events or abnormalities within the system involved. Each Medigraph Chart explains the causes (where known), shows the symptoms, explains current treatments, describes the complications that can occur and instructs in prevention (or lessening of impact).

In connection with the encyclopedic entries pertaining to specific medical conditions, this edition of *Fishbein's Illustrated Medical and Health Encyclopedia* makes available an original and unified feature in the form of discussions with medical consultants. To enrich and supplement the encyclopedic entries, collaborating medical and surgical authorities have contributed articles pertaining to their respective fields. Consulting discussions cover such topics as pregnancy, childbirth, postnatal care; infectious diseases of childhood and later life; allergies and skin disorders; heart, blood and digestive diseases; arthritis, rheumatism and gout; nutrition and diet for health and disease; old age and its problems; nervous and mental disorders; as well as many other topics. These are unified under the alphabetic sequence of the encyclopedic entries.

Public awareness of the tremendous expansion in medical knowledge is truly staggering. Newly discovered knowledge about conditions that affect the human body is constantly disseminated by features in mass circulating magazines and television programs. Medical background information of this nature is useful to the extent that it is based on scientific facts and related to specific medical conditions. To assure scientific accuracy and international viewpoint, this edition includes backgrounds in medical science from the *Mind Alive Encyclopedia.*

These are unified within the alphabetic framework following a pertinent medical entry. The reader seeking full, frank, authoritative information can now uncover fascinating scientific backgrounds that enlarge his or her understanding of specific medical subjects.

At the end of some encyclopedic articles you may see cross references preceded by one of these symbols ▶, ◆. These symbols precede the title of some unified feature that expands on the subject matter contained in the encyclopedic entry. They may refer to a consulting discussion by a leading medical specialist or to an article explaining the scientific background for some medical entry.

Here's a typical example. Suppose you have a question about *aging?* You naturally refer at once to the encyclopedia entry AGING and quickly obtain the information you seek. At the end of this encyclopedic entry, your attention is also called to the cross references bearing on the same subject as well as Medigraph Charts. You are then advised that a report on current research in the field follows the entry for CATARACTS. Should you want additional viewpoints by a qualified medical specialist, you will see cross references at the end of the encyclopedic entry preceded by the symbol ▶ which indicates a consulting discussion: a signed article by a distinguished medical authority pertaining to the subject AGING. Should you want to expand your knowledge of the subject, simply refer to the articles following the symbol ◆ which indicates a Medical Science Profile bearing on the topic AGING.

Similarly, if you have a question about the *adrenal gland,* then just refer to the encyclopedic entry ADRENAL GLAND under its alphabetic placement. After reading the entry, you again note cross references bearing on the same subject (such as ACTH; ADRENAL GLAND DISORDERS, etc.) as well as the Medigraph Charts ADDISON'S DISEASE, CUSHING'S SYNDROME and HYPOGLYCEMIA. Then you note cross references to a consulting discussion (▶) by a specialist of the adrenal glands (endocrine glands) and another discussion pertaining to the adrenal glands and skin. Following that you may want to refer to Medical Science Profiles (◆) Master Glands of the Human Body and (◆) Controlling the Cell System.

This unified editorial concept may be compared with a modern medical diagnostic and consultation service. Every specialty is brought into play. With the aid of these cross references, you broaden and deepen your understanding of the topic that interests you. Indeed, many readers seek out the unified features for sheer reading interest. A complete list of these features and their page numbers is in the Table of Contents starting on page xiii.

This work is not intended to substitute in any way for care by a physician. When remedies are mentioned, dosages are not supplied simply because any remedy that is capable of accomplishing an effect is just as likely to be harmful if given in wrong dosage. Self-diagnosis can be dangerous. The purpose of this book is, therefore, to be helpful to the physician, for it has long been established that an informed patient is more cooperative than one who is left in complete doubt as to what is going on.

A work of this nature involving so many different areas of medical practice must strive for factual accuracy. To assure such accuracy, we were fortunate in having the assistance of an outstanding group of medical authorities. At the invitation of Dr. Morris Fishbein, they contributed signed articles pertaining to their special areas of medicine. We are grateful to have had this cooperation which gave us the confidence to complete this Unified Edition following the concepts outlined by Dr. Morris Fishbein.

It is published now as a monument to a great figure in the field of medicine and medical writing; one who spent a lifetime challenging outmoded ideas, fighting off imposters, resisting unscientific change and clarifying the relationship of medicine to man.

H. S. STUTTMAN, INC.
Publishers

**VERNAL G. CAVE, M.D.**
Director, Bureau of Venereal Disease Control, Department of Health, New York City.

**J. DUDLEY CHAPMAN, D.O.**
Editor in Chief, *The Osteopathic Physician,* North Madison, O.

**ELIOT CORDAY, M.D.**
Cedars of Lebanon Hospital Division, Los Angeles, Calif.

**ISRAEL DAVIDSOHN, M.D.**
Director, Department of Experimental Pathology, Mount Sinai Hospital Medical Center, Chicago.

**UGO DEL TORTO, M.D.**
Director, Istituto di Clinica Ortopedica e Traumatologica, Universita di Napoli. Naples, Italy.

**THOMAS A. DOXIADIS, M.D.**
Former Chief of Medicine "Evangelismos" Medical Center, Athens, Greece.

**EUGENE M. FARBER, M.D.**
Professor and Chairman, Department of Dermatology, Stanford University Medical Center, Stanford, Calif.

**FRANKLIN R. FITCH, M.D.**
Professor of Dermatology Emeritus, Northwestern University Medical School; Director Emeritus, Institute for Sex Education, Chicago.

**RICHARD H. FREYBERG, M.D.**
Emeritus Director of Rheumatic Diseases, Hospital for Special Surgery, New York City; Consultant, internal medicine and rheumatic diseases, Scarsdale, N.Y.

**ROBERT B. GREENBLATT, M.D.**
Professor of Endocrinology, Medical College of Georgia, Augusta, Ga.

**E. DORINDA LOEFFEL, M.D.**
Assistant Professor of Dermatology, Stanford University Medical Center, Stanford, Calif.

**MARY HEWITT LOVELESS, M.D.**
Formerly Associate Professor Clinical Medicine (Allergy), Cornell University Medical College (New York Hospital), Westport, Conn.

**JULES H. MASSERMAN, M.D.**
Professor Emeritus, Psychiatry and Urology, Northwestern University; Honorary Life President, International Association for Social Psychiatry. Chicago.

**MARGARET A. OHLSON, PH.D.**

Author of "Experimental and Therapeutic Dietetics"; former Director of Nutrition Services, University Hospital and Professor of Internal Medicine, State University of Iowa College of Medicine, Iowa City. Seattle, Wash.

**SIR GEORGE PICKERING**

Master, Pembroke College, Oxford, England.

**PREBEN PLUM, M.D.**

Professor, University Clinic of Pediatrics, Rigshospitalet, Copenhagen, Denmark.

**HOWARD A. RUSK, M.D.**

Professor and Chairman, Department of Rehabilitation Medicine, New York University School of Medicine, New York City.

**ROBERT N. RUTHERFORD, M.D.**

Obstetrics, Gynecological Surgery and Fertility Clinic, Seattle, Wash.

**HANS SEYLE, M.D.**

Professor and Director, Institute of Experimental Medicine and Surgery, University of Montreal.

**MICHAEL B. SHIMKIN, M.D.**

Professor of Community Medicine and Oncology, University of California, San Diego. La Jolla, Calif.

**N. W. SHOCK, PH.D.**

Chief, Gerontology Research Center, Baltimore City Hospitals, Baltimore, Md.

**WILLIAM A. R. THOMSON, M.D.**

Former Editor, *The Practitioner,* London, England.

**EUGENE J. TAYLOR**

Adjunct Professor, Department of Rehabilitation Medicine, New York University School of Medicine, New York City.

**C. RAYMOND ZEISS, M.D.**

Major, USAF, MC, former Chief of Allergy-Immunology, U.S. Air Force Regional Hospital, Carswell AFB, Texas; Assistant Professor, Department of Medicine, Northwestern University Medical School, Chicago.

**FREDERICK P. ZUSPAN, M.D.**

Former Chairman, Department of Obstetrics and Gynecology, Chicago Lying-in Hospital, University of Chicago; Professor and Chairman, Department of Obstetrics and Gynecology, Ohio State University, Columbus.

**CONTRIBUTORS**

| | |
|---|---|
| IRVIN BLOCK | ELAINE LANDRY |
| FREDERIC DAMRAU, M.D. | HELENE MACLEAN |
| ARTHUR S. FREESE, M.D. | BARBARA MILBAUER |
| ARTHUR LAMIRANDE | EDWARD ROSENBERG |

**PRODUCTION EDITOR**
MAUREEN REHNBERG GARDELLA

**EDITORIAL ASSISTANT**
ELAINE LANDRY

**ANATOMICAL DRAWINGS**
LEONARD DANK
Medical Illustration Studio—St. Luke's Hospital, New York

**MEDIGRAPH CHARTS**
GEORGE E. PALEY, M.D. HERBERT C. ROSENTHAL
In collaboration with Graphics Institue, Inc.

**LAYOUT AND DESIGN**
MAUREEN REHNBERG GARDELLA

# CONTENTS

## VOLUME 1

**ABASIA** to **AGUE**

### MEDICAL RESEARCH REPORTS


Common "Gas Pain" Complaint Due to faulty Motility, Not Excess Amount ........ 36
Acupuncture Results Achieved Through Autonomic Nervous System ........ 64
Possible Hazard to Heart Function From Aerosols ........ 110
Participation in the Decision Important in Relocation of the Elderly .. 114


### MEDICAL SCIENCE PROFILES


Addiction's Vicious Circle ........ 66
The Child In Society ........ 80
Who Is the Adolescent? ........ 93


### MEDIGRAPH CHARTS


Acne ........ 55
Acromegaly and Giantism ........ 58
Addison's Disease ........ 72
Bronchial Adenoma ........ 75


### PHOTO STORIES


Accident Prevention ........ 43
Acupuncture ........ 61


### CONSULTING DISCUSSIONS


Aging ........ 114


### COLOR PLATES


Your Body and How It Functions ........ preceding Sites of Pain
Sites of Pain ........ Opposite 33


## VOLUME 2

**AINHUM** to **APOPLEXY**

### MEDICAL RESEARCH REPORTS


Healthy Lungs May Immunize Themselves Against Moderate Photochemical Smog ........ 148
Alcoholism Permanently Damages Liver in Spite of Nutritious Diet ... 158
New Advances in Allergy Sensitivity Testing, Immunotherapy and Diagnosis ........ 179
Excessive Intake of Vitamin C May Result in Anemia ........ 229

Interaction Between Medication and Anesthetics Investigated .......... 232
Studies Probe Possible Manufacture of Artificial Antibodies .......... 262
Chronic Prolonged Antihistamine Use May Cause Neuromuscular Disorder 264
New Noninvasive Technique Measures Narrowing of Arteries ....... 282

## MEDICAL SCIENCE PROFILES

A Better Life or Utter Chaos? ..... 148
How Nature Gets the Waste Away .. 161
The Body's Chemical Crutches .... 169
Another's Poison ............... 180
Scaling the Heights ............. 189
After the Egg .................. 199
Where Does Life Begin? .......... 218
Barriers Against Pain ........... 233
The Search for the Magic Bullet .... 256
Surgery Becomes Antiseptic ....... 267
Problem Personalities ............ 272

## MEDIGRAPH CHARTS

Alcoholism .................... 159
Amebiasis and Amebic Dysentery .. 197
Drug Abuse: Amphetamines ...... 211
Aneurysms .................... 239
Anthracosis and Asbestosis ........ 249
Anthrax ...................... 251

## PHOTO STORIES

Anaphylaxis .................. 215

## COLOR PLATES

Nervous System .......... Opposite 171

# VOLUME 3

## APPENDECTOMY to BLIND SPOT

## MEDICAL RESEARCH REPORTS

Needle Aspiration Treatment Effective for Septic Arthritis ......... 298
Lung-Damaging Asbestos Fibers Detected by Electron Microscopy ... 300
Ascorbic Acid Inhibits Rhinovirus Replication .................... 302
Steroid Treatment Appears Safe for Pregnant Asthmatics ............ 309
New Gallstone-Dissolving Drug May Also Reverse Atherosclerosis ..... 312
Single-Injection Contraceptive Effective for 12 Weeks ............. 377
Commonly Used Drug May Cause Serious Birth Defects ............ 399

## MEDICAL SCIENCE PROFILES

Bacteria—Agents of Decay ........ 324
The Families of Man ............ 355
How Large a Family? ............ 377
Born With a Problem ............ 399
Eyes to See With ............... 414

## MEDIGRAPH CHARTS

Appendicitis and Peritonitis ....... 284
Arteriosclerosis ................. 295

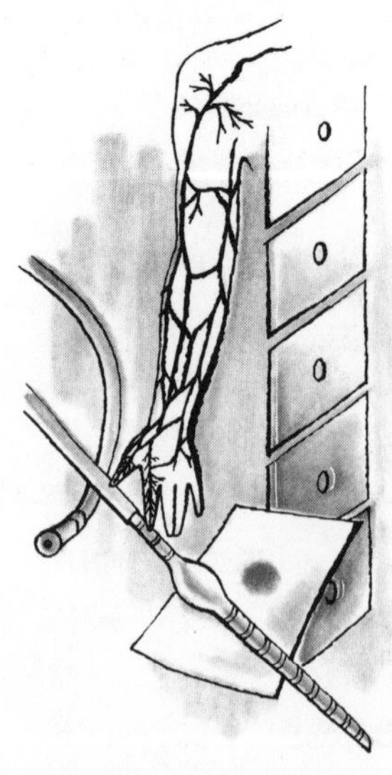

Drug Abuse: Barbiturates . . . . . . . . . 342
Bell's Palsy . . . . . . . . . . . . . . . . . . . . 365
Beriberi . . . . . . . . . . . . . . . . . . . . . . 367

**PHOTO STORIES**

Asthma . . . . . . . . . . . . . . . . . . . . . . . 305
Hair Transplant for Baldness . . . . . . 335

**CONSULTING DISCUSSIONS**

Wasp and Bee Sting Allergies . . . . . 349

**COLOR PLATES**

Birth, Development and Growth . . . . . . . . . . . . . . . . Opposite 309

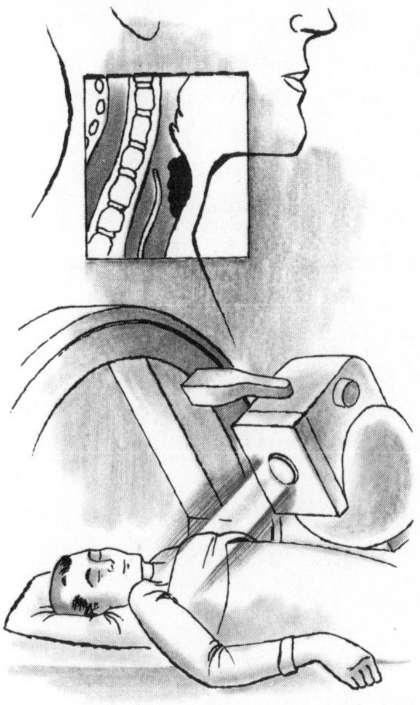

## VOLUME 4

### BLISTER BEETLE to CARCINOMA

**MEDICAL RESEARCH REPORTS**

Brain Researchers Create Nerve and Muscle Cell Connection . . . . . . . . . 477
Advanced Cancers Halted and Improved by New Combinations of Drugs . . . . . . . . . . . . . . . . . . . . 489
Heavy Coffee Drinking Not a Cause of Heart Disease in the Healthy Adult . . . . . . . . . . . . . . . . . . . . . . . 523
Point of Origin of Malignant Cells Ascertained by New Lab Technique 528
Rare Bone Cancer Responds to Female Hormone Therapy . . . . . . . . . 529

**MEDICAL SCIENCE PROFILES**

Life Blood . . . . . . . . . . . . . . . . . . . . . 425
What Type of Blood? . . . . . . . . . . . 458
How Do You Know? . . . . . . . . . . . . 477
How Nature Draws Breath . . . . . . . . 496
Cancer—Rogue Cells . . . . . . . . . . . 529

**MEDIGRAPH CHARTS**

Botulism . . . . . . . . . . . . . . . . . . . . . . 471
Brain Tumors . . . . . . . . . . . . . . . . . . 485
Breast Cancer . . . . . . . . . . . . . . . . . . 488
Bronchial Asthma . . . . . . . . . . . . . . . 505
Bronchiectasis . . . . . . . . . . . . . . . . . . 507
Bronchitis . . . . . . . . . . . . . . . . . . . . . 509
Buerger's Disease . . . . . . . . . . . . . . . 513
Bursitis . . . . . . . . . . . . . . . . . . . . . . . 521
Cancers of the Cervix and Uterus . . 537
Cancer of the Colon and Rectum . . . 539
Carbuncles, Furuncles and Folliculitis 557

**PHOTO STORIES**

Blood Processing . . . . . . . . . . . . . . . 455
Burn Treatment . . . . . . . . . . . . . . . . 515
Cancer Detection and Treatment . . . 543

**CONSULTING DISCUSSIONS**

The Blood and Its Diseases . . . . . . . 435
Cancer . . . . . . . . . . . . . . . . . . . . . . . . 540

**COLOR PLATES**

Blood and Lymph . . . . . . . . Opposite 447

## VOLUME 5

### CARDIAC to CLUBFOOT

**MEDICAL RESEARCH REPORTS**

Nonsurgical Treatment for Cataracts May Evolve from New Investigations . . . . . . . . . . . . . . . . . . . . . . . 572
Scientists Investigate Fetal Brain Damage Caused by Asphyxia During Pregnancy . . . . . . . . . . . . . 590

Some Cancer Chemotherapy May Increase Second Cancer Risk ..... 599
Plant-Derived Chemical Compound Shows Promise as Anticancer Drug 600
Antibody Production Based on Inherited Genetic Capability .......... 671

## MEDICAL SCIENCE PROFILES

A Guide for Careers ............ 562
The Cellular Units of Life ........ 580
Birth of a Child ................ 608
The Helpful Halogens ........... 657
Chromosomes—The Body's Blueprints ........................ 672
The Beat of the Blood ........... 684

## MEDIGRAPH CHARTS

Cataracts ...................... 571
Celiac Disease ................. 579
Cerebral Palsy ................. 589
Chagas' Disease ................ 597
Chickenpox ..................... 603
Cholera ........................ 667
Cirrhosis of the Liver ........... 693

## PHOTO STORIES

Cataract Surgery ............... 573
Cerebral Palsy ................. 591

## CONSULTING DISCUSSIONS

The Child ...................... 621

## COLOR PLATES

Circulatory System ....... Opposite 585

# VOLUME 6

## COAGULATION
to
## DEOXYRIBONUCLEIC ACID

## MEDICAL RESEARCH REPORTS

New Chemical in Nose Drops Reduces Cold Symptoms ........ 701
Dye-Light Treatment of Herpes Sores Found to be Ineffective ..... 704
Beating Heart Shown by New Scanning System ............... 735
Soft Contact Lenses Used in Treating Burned Eyes ........... 741
New Drugs Studied for Corneal Herpes Therapy ................ 751
New Storage Medium Maintains Freshness of Corneas for a Week .. 752
Nitroglycerin May Reduce Damage to Heart Muscle Following Severe Attack .................. 757
Mucus Transport Stimulant Benefits Cystic Fibrosis Patients .......... 784
Various Sugars Evaluated for Contributions to Tooth Decay .... 819
Decay-Causing Bacteria Transmitted to Infants by Mothers ........... 819
Adhesive Sealant Is Effective Tooth Decay Preventive ......... 830

## MEDICAL SCIENCE PROFILES

Diseases of Childhood ............ 707
Fate and the Human Egg ......... 717
The Learning Game .............. 724
Houses for the Sick ............. 743
Network of the Nerves ........... 761
Cracking Open the Cell ........... 785
The Point of Death .............. 803
Battle Against Decay ............ 820

## MEDIGRAPH CHARTS

Drug Abuse: Cocaine ............ 698
Cold Sores ...................... 703
Congenital Heart Disease ......... 734
Conjunctivitis ................... 737
Contact Dermatitis and Drug Reactions ...................... 739

Cretinism and Myxedema ......... 770
Cushing's Syndrome .............. 779

PHOTO STORIES

Cryosurgery .................... 774
Cystic Fibrosis .................. 781
Hearing Tests .................... 797
Dental Research ................. 828

MEDIGRAPH CHARTS

Deviated Septum ................ 854
Diabetes ......................... 857
Diphtheria ...................... 953

CONSULTING DISCUSSIONS

Planning the Diet ............... 878
Digestive Diseases ............... 916

COLOR PLATES

Digestive System ......... Opposite 861

## VOLUME 7

**DEPILATORY** to **DRESSING**

MEDICAL RESEARCH REPORTS

DES Effects on Offspring Investigated ........................ 851
Hormone Useful in Diabetes Therapy Does Not Impair Human Blood Clotting ...................... 864
Fluid Removal Facilitated by New Filtration System ............... 875
Weight Fluctuation Increases Risk of Gallstones in Obese Patients ... 903

MEDICAL SCIENCE PROFILES

When Life Is "Not Worth Living" .. 837
Skin: The Perfect Wrapper ........ 843
Looking for Trouble ............. 868
Burning Up the Food We Eat ...... 907
Doctor and Patient ............... 962

## VOLUME 8

**DROPSY** to **EUGENICS**

MEDICAL RESEARCH REPORTS

High Histamine Levels in Eczema Patients Increase Risk of Bacterial Infection ...................... 1014
Enzyme Deficiency Responsible for One Type of Emphysema ........ 1038
Explanation Offered for Widespread Bacterial Endocarditis in Heroin Addicts ....................... 1045
Laboratory Test Determines Blood Levels of Medication ............ 1098

MEDICAL SCIENCE PROFILES

The Intricate Ear ................ 995
The Fuel of Life ................. 1006
Why the Egg Becomes a Chicken ... 1022
The Flame of Life ............... 1072
Health and the Environment ...... 1080
Diseases on the Map .............1090
The Shape of Human Beings to Come 1103

MEDIGRAPH CHARTS

Eclampsia and Preeclampsia ....... 1005
Ectopic Pregnancy ............... 1012
Emphysema .................... 1039
Encephalitis .................... 1041
Subacute Bacterial Endocarditis .... 1044
Epilepsy ....................... 1097
Diseases of the Esophagus ........ 1101

PHOTO STORIES

Drug Abuse .................... 975

Drug Withdrawal . . . . . . . . . . . . . . . . 981
Training Emotionaly Disturbed . . . . 1032

**CONSULTING DISCUSSIONS**

The Endocrine Glands . . . . . . . . . . . . 1046

**COLOR PLATES**

Endocrine System . . . . . . . . Opposite 999

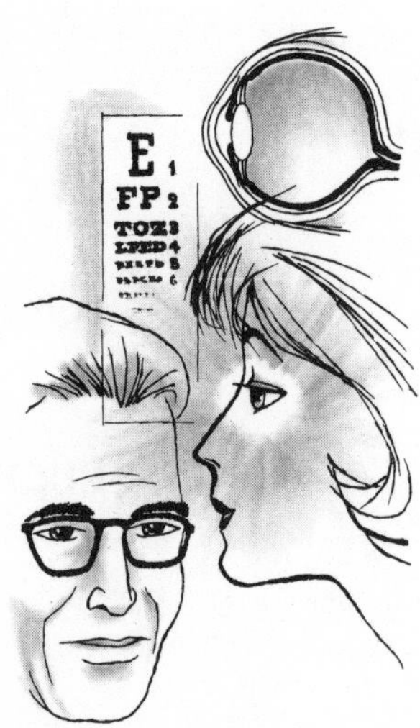

## VOLUME 9

**EUNUCH**

to

**FIRST AID**

**MEDICAL RESEARCH REPORTS**

Bone Cancer Survival Rates Increased by New Combination Therapy . . . . 1120
New Device Inserted in the Eye Delivers Continuous Flow of Medication . . . . . . . . . . . . . . . . . . . 1150
Scientists Isolate Two Proteins Responsible for Fever in Humans . . 1213

**MEDICAL SCIENCE PROFILES**

In the Name of Progress . . . . . . . . . . 1112
After the Energy Has Gone . . . . . . . 1121
Competing for the Prize . . . . . . . . . . 1135
Road Accident! . . . . . . . . . . . . . . . . . 1243

**MEDIGRAPH CHARTS**

Fibroid Tumor . . . . . . . . . . . . . . . . . 1215
Fibromyositis . . . . . . . . . . . . . . . . . . 1217

**PHOTO STORIES**

Exercise Equipment . . . . . . . . . . . . . . 1132

**CONSULTING DISCUSSIONS**

The Human Eye . . . . . . . . . . . . . . . . . 1151

## VOLUME 10

**FISH**

to

**GONORRHEA**

**MEDICAL RESEARCH REPORTS**

Experiment Reveals Fluoride in Food Affords Less Tooth Protection Than Fluoride in Water . . . . . . . . . . 1266
New Electromagnetic Technique Regenerates Bone Tissue . . . . . . . . . 1288
Dissolving of Gallstones by Bile Acid May Eliminate Need for Surgery . . 1314
Combination Medication More Effective in Dissolving Gallstones . . 1314
Antibody-Rich Preparation May Impede Hepatitis B Immunity . . . . 1316
Calf Virus Used to Test Infantile Gastroenteritis May Become Basis of Immunizing Vaccine . . . . . . . . . . 1320
New Test Identifies Cystic Fibrosis Carriers . . . . . . . . . . . . . . . . . . . . . . 1341
New Technique Analyzes Mother's Blood for Fetal Defects . . . . . . . . . 1342
Tissue Destroying Enzyme Linked to Gingivitis . . . . . . . . . . . . . . . . . . 1368
Specific Agent Responsible for Immunological Failure in Kidney Disorder . . . . . . . . . . . . . . . . . . . . 1380

**MEDICAL SCIENCE PROFILES**

Bloodsuckers and Hangers-On . . . . . 1259
Our Daily Bread . . . . . . . . . . . . . . . 1270
The Chemicals We Eat . . . . . . . . . . . 1279
Winter Sports . . . . . . . . . . . . . . . . . . 1293
Parasites and Scavengers . . . . . . . . . 1302
Genes—Life's Changing Stereotypes 1322
The Needs of the Aged . . . . . . . . . . . 1343
Why Do We Grow Old? . . . . . . . . . . 1362
Master Glands of the Human Body . 1370

**MEDIGRAPH CHARTS**

Flu . . . . . . . . . . . . . . . . . . . . . . . . . . 1255

Fractures and Dislocations ........ 1289
Fungus Infections of the Skin ..... 1301
Gallstones ...................... 1315
Gastritis ........................ 1319
German Measles ................ 1352
Glaucoma ...................... 1379
Drug Abuse: Sniffing of Glue, Solvents, Aerosols, Anesthetics ... 1382
Gonorrhea ..................... 1385

### PHOTO STORIES

Control and Prevention of Flu ..... 1256
Genetic Analysis ................ 1331
Aging Research ................. 1354

## VOLUME 11

**GOODPASTURE'S SYNDROME**

to

**HEEL**

### MEDICAL RESEARCH REPORTS

Stunted Children Benefit from Wide Distribution of Growth Hormone .. 1395
Cellular Studies Could Promote Improved Allergy Testing and Treatment ..................... 1442
Human Heart Cells Grown in Laboratory ..................... 1462
Heart Attack Damage May Be Monitored and Controlled by New Techniques ..................... 1470
Program to Investigate New Synthetics for Artificial Organs ......... 1485

### MEDICAL SCIENCE PROFILES

The Price of Health ............. 1391
Health and Wealth .............. 1447
Making Sense of Sounds .......... 1455
Ten Thousand Miles Around the Human Heart ................. 1463

### MEDIGRAPH CHARTS

Gout .......................... 1388
Hansen's Disease ............... 1439
Hay Fever ..................... 1441
Heart Failure .................. 1473
Heat Stroke .................... 1523

### PHOTO STORIES

Head Injuries .................. 1446
Hearing Aids ................... 1453
Heart Surgery .................. 1476
Mechanical Devices for the Heart .. 1481
Intensive Coronary Care Unit ..... 1501

### CONSULTING DISCUSSIONS

The Health of Women ........... 1397
Diseases of the Heart and Circulation 1486

### COLOR PLATES

Skin and Hair ........... Opposite 1413

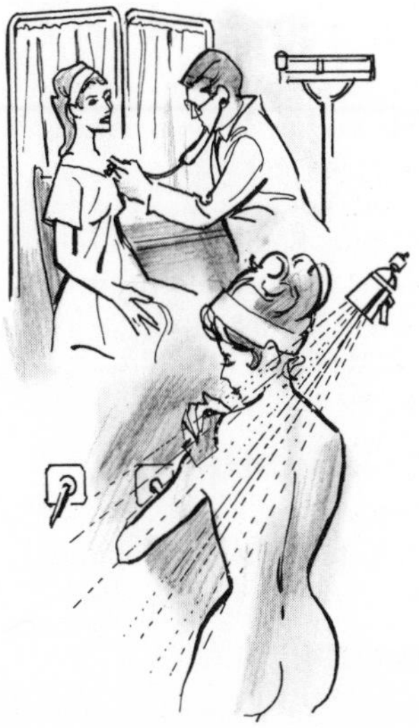

## VOLUME 12

**HEIGHT**

to

**ILEUM**

### MEDICAL RESEARCH REPORTS

Vaccine Immunization Against Hepatitis Found Safe, Effective, in Chimp Studies ............... 1542
Further Substantiation of Dane Particle as Viral Cause of Hepatitis B 1542
Family History May Be Clue to Cancer Proneness ............... 1544
Effects of Hypertension Drugs on Timed Responses Investigated .... 1553

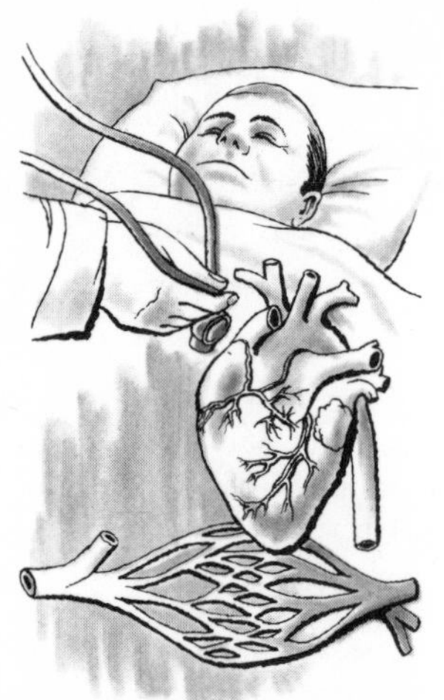


Pressure Therapy Yields 90 Percent Survival of Newborns with Respiratory Distress Syndrome ... 1606
New Diagnostic Technique Advances Early Treatment of Parathyroid Disease ... 1628
Hypothermia Enables Safe Removal of Brain Tumor ... 1643
Hypothermia Makes Heart Surgery Possible for Delicate Infants ... 1643
Crohn's Disease Distinguished by Distinctive Serum Enzyme ... 1662


## MEDICAL SCIENCE PROFILES


Reaching for Maturity ... 1526
Controlling the Cell System ... 1583
Hotels for Healing ... 1593
Enough Is As Good As a Feast ... 1598
Acids and Alkalis ... 1608
The Right to Health ... 1618
Hypnosis: Magnetism or Medicine? ... 1634
Awareness of the Unconscious ... 1646
Tracing Characteristics ... 1654


## MEDIGRAPH CHARTS


Hemophilia ... 1535
Hemorrhoids and Fissures ... 1539
Hepatitis ... 1541
Drug Abuse: Heroin ... 1547
Hiatus Hernia ... 1549
High Blood Pressure ... 1551
Histoplasmosis ... 1571
Hives ... 1573
Hodgkin's Disease ... 1575
Hookworm ... 1581
Hyperparathyroidism ... 1627
Hypertensive Heart Disease ... 1629
Hyperthyroidism ... 1631
Hypoglycemia ... 1639
Ileitis ... 1661


## CONSULTING DISCUSSIONS


Hypertension and Vascular Disease ... 1553


# VOLUME 13

## IMBECILE to INSECTICIDES

## MEDICAL RESEARCH REPORTS


White Cells in Mother's Milk May Cause Graft-Vs.-Host Disease ... 1664
Common Virus Links Birth Defects to Mother's Faulty Immunity ... 1664
Cause of Rare Immune-Deficiency Disease Discovered by Cancer Scientists ... 1665
Antibodies Responsible for Suppressing Hypersensitivity Are Identified 1684
Fumes From Heated Adhesive on Labels May Cause Meatwrappers' Asthma ... 1693
Newborns Capable of Taste Distinction and Preference ... 1700
Doctors and Patients Alerted to Need for Fire Ant Sting Desensitization .. 1799
Insect Sting Sensitivity Detected by Improved Test ... 1800


## MEDICAL SCIENCE PROFILES


A Shot in the Arm ... 1678
Dangers on the Job ... 1694
A Child's First Year ... 1702
Bring Out Your Dead! ... 1716
The Science Behind the Cure ... 1751
The Problems of Infertility ... 1761
Humanity Against Itself ... 1774
The Child in the Family ... 1781
First Steps to Childhood ... 1789


## MEDIGRAPH CHARTS


Impetigo ... 1687
Inguinal and Other Abdominal Hernias ... 1771


## PHOTO STORIES


Infectious Microorganisms ... 1712

**CONSULTING DISCUSSIONS**

Immunology and the Allergic Diseases ..... 1665
Infectious Diseases ..... 1722


# VOLUME 14

## INSOMNIA to LUPUS VULGARIS


**MEDICAL RESEARCH REPORTS**

Two Drugs Evaluated for Lupus Nephritis Therapy ..... 1865
Wearable Artificial Kidney Being Developed ..... 1879
Dietary Supplement of Synthesized Acids Improves Condition of Kidney Patients ..... 1880
Tiny Organisms May Be Nucleus of Bladder Stone Formations ..... 1883
Leukemia Remission Achieved by Bone Marrow Transplant from Twin ..... 1909
New Test May Predict Effectiveness of Drugs Used in Leukemia Therapy 1909
Component in Leukemic Cells Provides Basis for Effectiveness of Drug Treatment ..... 1910
Leukemia Relapse Predictable Through Bone Marrow Culture Test ..... 1910
Improved Dosage Regulation of Cyclophosphamide Based on New Tests ..... 1938

**MEDICAL SCIENCE PROFILES**

Tests of Human Intelligence ..... 1807
Rays to Kill or Cure ..... 1827
Tracing the Pathways of Life ..... 1838
The Body's Purifying Plant ..... 1865
Extensions of the Human Eye ..... 1897

**MEDIGRAPH CHARTS**

Intestinal Obstruction ..... 1818
Iritis ..... 1825
Kidney and Urinary Tract Stones .. 1882
Lead Poisoning ..... 1893
Leptospirosis ..... 1904
Leukemia ..... 1907
Leukoplakia ..... 1912
Lice and Scabies ..... 1915
Drug Abuse: LSD ..... 1929
Lung Abscess ..... 1931
Lung Cancer ..... 1933
Lupus Erythematosus ..... 1937

**PHOTO STORIES**

Sterile Room ..... 1836
Kidney Dialysis ..... 1875

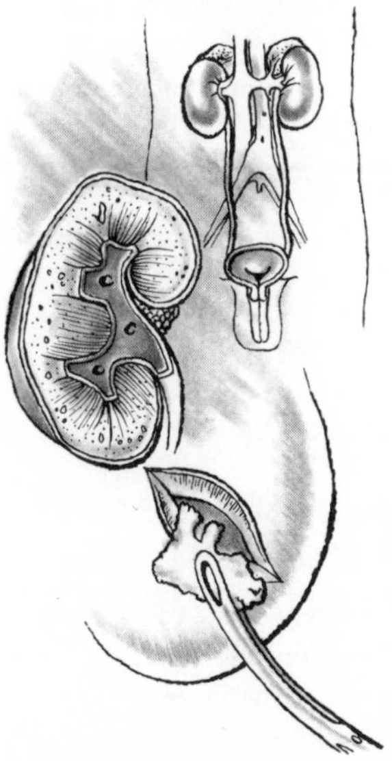

# VOLUME 15

## LYME DISEASE to MUSCULAR DYSTROPHY


**MEDICAL RESEARCH REPORTS**

Screening Tests of Human Immune System May Indicate Presence of Cancer ..... 1940
Human Lymph Cancer Cell Cultures Grown by New Lab Technique ... 1942
Malaria Parasites Observed and Filmed by New Electro-optical System ..... 1947
Correction of Muscular Imbalance May Become New Orthodontic Procedure ..... 1948

Personality Change Can Result From Long-Term Heavy Marijuana Use . 1960
Cancer Recurrence Reduced by Postoperative Three-Drug Chemotherapy ................ 1963
Chemical Changes in Brain Cells Linked to Memory Formation .... 1994
Faulty Immunity May Explain Predisposition to Fungal Meningitis .................... 1998
New Program Stimulates Communication Endeavors by Severely Retarded Children .............. 2013
Recently Isolated Virus May Be Cause of Mononucleosis ......... 2060
Molecular Defect in Worm Muscle May Be Clue to Human Dystrophies 2076
Newly Isolated Biochemical May Aid in Clarifying Muscular Dystrophy . 2076

## MEDICAL SCIENCE PROFILES

Understanding the Sick in Mind .... 1951
Keeping Up with Disease ......... 1973
Life's Vital Membranes ........... 1985
Keeping a Balance ............... 2004
A Closer Look at Life ............ 2021
Rituals of Childbirth ............ 2044

## MEDIGRAPH CHARTS

Malaria ....................... 1945
Drug Abuse: Marijuana and Hashish 1959
Mastoiditis .................... 1965
Measles ....................... 1967
Ménière's Disease ............... 1995
Meningitis ..................... 1997
Menopause .................... 1999
Mercury Poisoning ............. 2015
Drug Abuse: Mescaline and Peyote . 2016
Migraine Headaches ............ 2054
Infectious Mononucleosis ......... 2059
Multiple Sclerosis .............. 2067
Mumps ...................... 2068

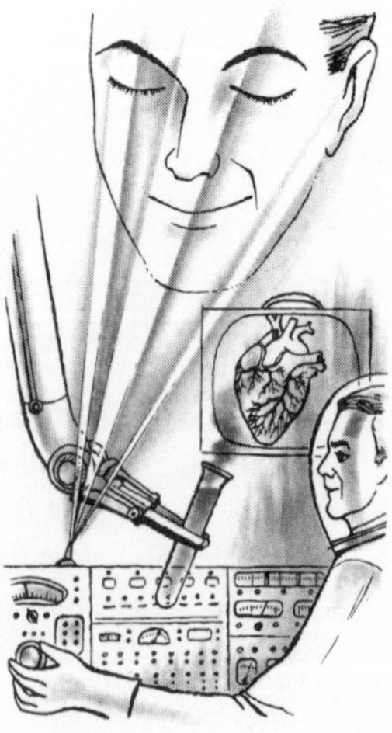

## PHOTO STORIES

Muscular Dystrophy ............. 2073

## CONSULTING DISCUSSIONS

Conquering the Climacteric ........ 2033

# VOLUME 16

## MUSHROOMS to ORINASE

## MEDICAL RESEARCH REPORTS

Early Diagnosis of Multiple Myeloma Made Possible by New Technique.. 2086
New Study Highlights Causes of Interstitial Nephritis ........... 2098
New Chemical Test Detects Niemann-Pick Disease Carriers ... 2126
Wide-Ranging Research Program Studies Harmful Effects of Noise .. 2130
Heart Attack Damage Made Visible by Scanning .................. 2145
New Test Alerts Doctors to Rejection of Heart Transplant ........... 2213
Greater Transplant Success Seen with Rapid Typing Technique .... 2214

## MEDICAL SCIENCE PROFILES

Change, Modification and Decay ... 2078
The Nervous System ........... 2105
Processing the Information ........ 2120
The Science of Sound ........... 2131
Radiation in the Service of Humanity 2145
Vital Members of the Medical Team 2154
We Are What We Eat ........... 2172
The First Breath ............... 2184
Learning to Live Again ......... 2192

## MEDIGRAPH CHARTS

Myasthenia Gravis ............ 2085
Coronary Artery Disease (Myocardial Infarction) ........ 2088

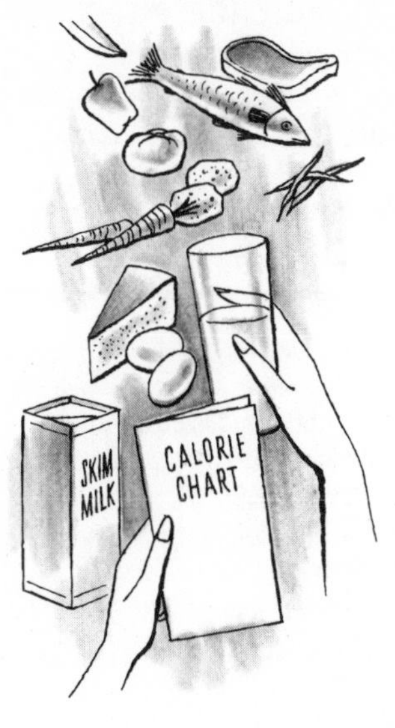


Nephritis ........................ 2097
Neuritis ........................ 2111
Neurocirculatory Asthenia ........ 2112
Orchitis ........................ 2209

**PHOTO STORIES**

Nuclear Medicine ................ 2141
Nursing Home .................. 2160
Eye Examination ................ 2201
Vision Aids .................... 2206

**COLOR PLATES**

Muscular System ....... Opposite 2103

## VOLUME 17

**ORTHODONTIA**

to

**PIMPLES**

**MEDICAL RESEARCH REPORTS**

Facial Bones of Monkeys Altered to Fit Existing Dentition ......... 2216
Orthodontic Widening of Upper Jaw Also Corrects Faulty Breathing ... 2216
Higher Adult Calcium Consumption Recommended to Forestall Osteoporosis .................. 2242
Measurement of Dental Pain Achieved by Use of Electrodes ... 2260
Pancreatic Cells on Artificial Capillaries Continue to Produce Insulin . 2268
New Medications Evaluated for Elimination of Side Effects ....... 2288
Sterile Environment Protects Vulnerable Hospital Patients ...... 2299
Hepatitis B in the Newborn Prevented by Antibody Treatment . 2309
Connection Established Between Inflamed Gums and Bone Loss .... 2310

**MEDICAL SCIENCE PROFILES**

The Active Element of Oxygen .... 2249
Pain—The Body's Warning System . 2260
Living Together ................ 2275
Agents of Disease and Decay ...... 2290
Microbes Versus the Body ........ 2317
Medicine Through the Ages ...... 2326
A Time to Play ................ 2336
The Healing Knife .............. 2344

**MEDIGRAPH CHARTS**

Osteoarthritis .................. 2235
Osteomyelitis .................. 2237
Ovarian Infection ............... 2244
Cancer of the Pancreas .......... 2269
Pancreatitis .................... 2271
Parkinson's Disease ............ 2287
Pellagra ....................... 2301
Pericarditis .................... 2305
Peripheral Arteriosclerosis ........ 2311
Pernicious Anemia ............. 2313
Phlebitis ...................... 2333
Pilonidal Cyst ................. 2351

**PHOTO STORIES**

Orthodontia ................... 2217
Drug Manufacturing ............ 2324

**CONSULTING DISCUSSIONS**

Common Orthopedic Complaints ... 2222
Osteopathy ................... 2238

## VOLUME 18

**PINEAL GLAND**

to

**QUINTUPLETS**

**MEDICAL RESEARCH REPORTS**

Polychlorinated Biphenyl Food Levels Affect Pregnancies in Monkeys .... 2377

High Blood Pressure May Result from Deficiency of Prostaglandins . 2429
Psoriasis Studies Advanced by Skin-Grafted Mice ............. 2436
Photochemotherapy Clears Skin Lesions of Psoriasis Patients ...... 2438

**MEDICAL SCIENCE PROFILES**

Skin Sculpture .................. 2361
Maternal Home of the Unborn .... 2385
Pregnancy and Its Problems ...... 2398
Life Before Birth ............... 2407
Global Battle for Better Health .... 2422
Exploring the Mind .............. 2449
Up and Out of Childhood ........ 2459
Public Health .................. 2468
Against a Common Enemy ........ 2482

**MEDIGRAPH CHARTS**

Pinworm ...................... 2354
Pityriasis Rosea ................ 2358
Pleurisy ...................... 2369
Pneumonia ................... 2373
Poliomyelitis .................. 2375
Prostate Gland Enlargement—Cancer of the Prostate .......... 2431
Psoriasis ..................... 2437
Pulmonary Heart Disease ........ 2475

**PHOTO STORIES**

Premature Births ................ 2393
Preventive Medicine ............. 2418

**CONSULTING DISCUSSIONS**

Psychiatry ..................... 2439

## VOLUME 19

### RABBIT FEVER to SCRUB TYPHUS

**MEDICAL RESEARCH REPORTS**

Leukemia Survival Time Doubled by Total Body Irradiation ........ 2496
Salivary Gland Damage Is Side Effect of Head/Neck Radiation Therapy . 2497
New Diet Counteracts Radiation Enteritis ..................... 2497
Rheumatoid Arthritics Respond Well to New Combination Therapy .... 2566

**MEDICAL SCIENCE PROFILES**

Shaping Nature to Need .......... 2506
Animals and Sexual Reproduction .. 2527
The Start of a Cure .............. 2542
The Breath of Life .............. 2548
Schizophrenia's Disordered World .. 2617

**MEDIGRAPH CHARTS**

Rabies ........................ 2492
Raynaud's Disease ............... 2502
Rheumatic Fever ................ 2561
Rheumatic Heart Disease ......... 2563
Rheumatoid Arthritis ............ 2565
Rickets ....................... 2600
Rocky Mounted Spotted Fever .... 2605
Roundworm ................... 2607
Scarlet Fever .................. 2613
Schistosomiasis ................. 2615
Scleroderma .................. 2627

**PHOTO STORIES**

Rehabilitation .................. 2515
Rheumatoid Arthritis ............ 2575

**CONSULTING DISCUSSIONS**

Rehabilitation .................. 2512
The Rheumatic Diseases .......... 2567

**COLOR PLATES**

Respiratory System ...... Opposite 2517

## VOLUME 20

### SCURVY to STRETCH MARKS

**MEDICAL RESEARCH REPORTS**

Monkey Virus May Shed Light on Chickenpox and Shingles ........ 2654
Surgical Patients with Sickle Cell Anemia Need Special Anesthetic Management .................. 2667
Synthetic Hormone Effective in Hereditary Bone Disease ........ 2678
Successful New Speech Therapy Uses Computer-Based System ......... 2728

**MEDICAL SCIENCE PROFILES**

Shock Report .................. 2657
The Lively Machinery of Bone and Muscle ...................... 2679

The Twilight Zone .............. 2715
The Ability to Speak ............ 2733

## MEDIGRAPH CHARTS

Scurvy ........................ 2630
Seborrheic Dermatitis ............ 2632
Shingles ....................... 2655
Sickle Cell Anemia ............ 2666
Silicosis ....................... 2669
Hypogonadism and Simmonds' Disease ...................... 2670
Sinusitis ....................... 2673
Skin Cancer .................... 2712
Slipped Disc ................... 2721
Snake Bites .................... 2724
Sprains and Strains ............. 2751
Sterility ....................... 2754
Stomach Cancer ................ 2757

## PHOTO STORIES

Sickle Cell Anemia .............. 2664
Dermatologist .................. 2703
Speech Therapy ................. 2729
Stress Testing .................. 2763

## CONSULTING DISCUSSIONS

Sex and Sex Education .......... 2637
The Importance of Skin .......... 2688
Stress Without Distress .......... 2759

## COLOR PLATES

Skeletal System .......... Opposite 2655

# VOLUME 21

## STRICTURE to VACCINATION

## MEDICAL RESEARCH REPORTS

Long-Term Reduction of Blood Pressure Safe for Stroke Patients .. 2768
Significant Advances in Medical and Surgical Stroke Treatment ....... 2770
Congenital Cardiac Irregularity May Cause Sudden Infant Death Syndrome .................... 2779
New Test Alerts Doctors to Possibility of Sudden Infant Death .. 2779
New Alarm System Monitors Infant Breathing .................... 2780
Cellular Immunity Suppression May Explain Clinical Course of Syphilis 2796
"Feeding" Tay-Sachs Cells with Enzyme May Advance Treatment of the Disease ................ 2806
Fluoride Must Be Ingested from Infancy for Maximum Benefit to Children's Teeth ............... 2809
School-Administered Fluoride Tablets Lower Tooth Decay ...... 2810
New Telemetry Techniques Simplify Patient Monitoring ............. 2810
Cooley's Anemia Diagnosable in Fetus Using Aspiration Technique.. 2835
Pregnant Women Alerted to Danger of Toxoplasmosis Exposure ...... 2850
Tracers Detect Lengthy Survival of Toxoplasmosis Oocysts in Soil .... 2850
Computerized Donor Lists Facilitate Transfusions of Vital Blood Component ................... 2854
Visual Technique Replaces Surgery in Diagnosis of Kidney Tumors ... 2884
Some Cases of Urethritis Caused by Newly Isolated Bacterial Strain ... 2898
Antibiotic Taken Orally After Intercourse Prevents Chronic Bladder Infections .............. 2901
Tooth Decay May One Day Be Preventable by Vaccination ...... 2904

## MEDICAL SCIENCE PROFILES

Stroke ........................ 2770
On the Operating Table .......... 2784
Taste and Smell ................. 2800
People Under Stress ............. 2814

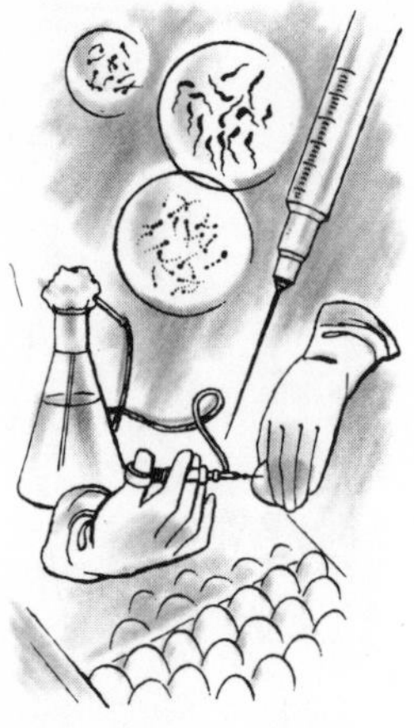

Detective Chemistry ............. 2825
The War Behind the Lines ........ 2856
Disease in the Tropics ............ 2869
The White Plague ............... 2878

## MEDIGRAPH CHARTS

Stroke ........................ 2769
Sty ............................ 2777
Syphilis ....................... 2795
Tapeworm ..................... 2799
Tay-Sachs Disease ............... 2807
Tetanus ....................... 2833
Thyroid Heart Disease ........... 2842
Acute Tonsillitis ................ 2847
Toxoplasmosis .................. 2851
Trench Mouth .................. 2863
Trichinosis .................... 2865
Trichomonas .................... 2866
Pulmonary Tuberculosis .......... 2877
Typhoid Fever ................. 2885
Ulcerative Colitis .............. 2889
Ulcers of the Digestive Tract ...... 2891
Undescended Testicles ............ 2895
Urinary Tract Tumors and Infections 2899

## COLOR PLATES

Special Sense Organs .... Opposite 2793

# 22

# VAGINA to ZYME INDEX

## MEDICAL RESEARCH REPORTS

Virus Isolated from Lab-Grown Human Leukemic Cells ......... 2926
Activated Form of Vitamin D Beneficial for Bone Lesions ...... 2961

## MEDICAL SCIENCE PROFILES

The Virus—Scourge of the Cell .... 2927
Vitamins—The Cornerstones of Health ....................... 2962
Open Secrets in an X-ray's Beam .. 2986

## MEDIGRAPH CHARTS

Hydrocele and Varicocele ......... 2907
Varicose Veins ................. 2909
Vitamin A Deficiency ............ 2958
Warts ......................... 2971
Whiplash Injury of the Neck ...... 2976
Whooping Cough ............... 2979
Yellow Fever .................. 2993

## PHOTO STORIES

Low Vision .................. 2933

## CONSULTING DISCUSSIONS

The Venereal Diseases ........... 2912
Vision Impairment ............. 2938

## COLOR PLATES

The Human Body in Anatomical Transparencies ......... Opposite 2995

PICTURE CREDITS .............. 2995
INDEX ........................ 3003

# ACKNOWLEDGMENTS

To maintain a high standard of accuracy and assure clarity in conveying technical information, the publishers requested the cooperation of medical and health foundations, research institutions and corporations identified with medical progress. The following organizations were most helpful in answering the many queries of our editors and writers and very generous in supplying current photographs whenever such illustrations were needed to supplement the text: AMERICAN CANCER SOCIETY; AMERICAN HEART ASSOCIATION; AMERICAN STERILIZER COMPANY; BECTON, DICKINSON AND COMPANY; BIOMEDICAL GRAPHIC COMMUNICATIONS; CITY OF HOPE; CYSTIC FIBROSIS FOUNDATION; DAHLBERG ELECTRONICS, INC.; EDWARDS LABORATORIES; GUNDERSON CLINIC, LTD.; JOHNSON & JOHNSON; THE LONDON COMPANY; MARION HEALTH AND SAFETY; METROPOLITAN LIFE; MILES LABORATORIES; NATIONAL FOUNDATION/MARCH OF DIMES; NEW YORK ASSOCIATION FOR THE BLIND; OHIO-NUCLEAR, INC.; PARKE, DAVIS & CO.; PERKIN-ELMER CORPORATION; SEARLE RADIOGRAPHICS, INC.; and SYNTEX LABORATORIES.

The publishers acknowledge their gratitude to these organizations for their genuine interest in this work. Special thanks are due to the staff at the NATIONAL INSTITUTES OF HEALTH in Bethesda, Maryland. They were most cooperative in familiarizing our staff with the results of their vast activities in each area of medical research.

H. S. STUTTMAN CO., INC.
*Publishers*

# Key to Derivation of Medical Terms

THESE medical combining forms, with a prefix or a suffix, or both, are those most commonly used in making medical words. **G** indicates those from the Greek; **L**, those from Latin. Properly Greek forms should be used only with Greek prefixes and suffixes; Latin, with Latin. A vowel, usually a, i, or o, is often needed for euphony.

## MEDICAL COMBINING FORMS

**Acr- (G)** *pertaining to extremity:* acrodermatitis, a dermatitis of the limbs.

**Aden- (G)** *pertaining to a gland:* adenitis, inflammation of a gland.

**Bio- (G)** *pertaining to life:* biopsy, inspection of living organism (or tissue).

**Bleph- (G)** *pertaining to eyelids:* blepharitis, inflammation of an eyelid.

**Cardi (G)** *pertaining to heart:* cardialgia, pain in the heart.

**Cephal- (G)** *pertaining to head:* cephalalgia, headache.

**Cheil- (G)** *pertaining to lip:* cheilitis, inflammation of the lip.

**Cheir- (G)** *pertaining to hand:* cheirospasm, writer's cramp.

**Chole- (G)** *pertaining to bile:* cholecyst, the gallbladder.

**Chondr- (G)** *pertaining to cartilage:* chondrectomy, removal of a cartilage.

**Cleid- (G)** *pertaining to clavicle:* cleidocostal, pertaining to clavicle and ribs.

**Colp- (G)** *pertaining to vagina:* colporrhagia, vaginal hemorrhage.

**Cost- (G)** *pertaining to rib:* costalgia, pain in the ribs.

**Crani- (L)** *pertaining to skull:* craniotomy, surgical opening in skull.

**Crypt- (G)** *pertaining to anything hidden:* cryptogenic, hidden or unknown origin.

**Cyst- (G)** *pertaining to fluid-containing sac:* cystitis, inflammation of bladder.

**Cyt- (G)** *pertaining to a cell:* cytometer, device for counting and measuring cells.

**Dacry- (G)** *pertaining to lachrymal glands:* dacryocyst, tear-sac.

**Derm-** or **dermat- (G)** *pertaining to skin:* dermatoid, skinlike.

**Encephal- (G)** *pertaining to brain:* encephalitis, inflammation of brain.

**Enter- (G)** *pertaining to intestine:* enteroptosis, falling of intestine.

**Galact- (G)** *pertaining to milk:* galactose, a milk sugar.

**Gastr- (G)** *pertaining to stomach:* gastrectomy, excision of the stomach.

**Gynec- (G)** *pertaining to woman:* gynecology, science of diseases of women.

**Hem-** or **hemat- (G)** *pertaining to blood:* hemopoiesis, forming blood.

**Hyster- (G)** *pertaining to uterus:* hysterectomy, excision of uterus.

**Kerat- (G)** *pertaining to horn, cornea:* keratitis, infammation of cornea.

**Kopr-** or **copr-** **(G)** *pertaining to feces:* coprolith, a fecal concretion.

**Leuk-** or **leuc-** **(G)** *pertaining to anything white:* leukocyte, white cell.

**Mer-** **(G)** *part:* merotomy, division into segments.

**Metr-** **(G)** *pertaining to uterus:* metritis, inflammation of uterus.

**My-** **(G)** *pertaining to muscle:* myoma, tumor made of muscular elements.

**Myc-** **(G)** *pertaining to fungi:* mycology, science and study of fungi.

**Neo-** **(G)** *new:* neoplasm, any new growth or formation.

**Neph-** **(G)** *pertaining to kidney:* nephrectomy, surgical excision of kidney.

**Odont-** **(G)** *pertaining to tooth:* odontology, dentistry.

**Omo-** **(G)** *pertaining to shoulder:* omohyoid, pertaining to shoulder and hyoid bone.

**Oö-** **(G)** *pertaining to egg:* oöcyte, original cell of egg.

**Oöphor-** **(G)** *pertaining to ovary:* oöphorectomy, removal of an ovary.

**Ophthalm-** **(G)** *pertaining to eye:* ophthalmometer, an instrument for measuring the eye.

**Oss-** **(L)** *pertaining to bone:* osseous, bony.

**Oste-** **(G)** *pertaining to bone:* osteitis, inflammation of a bone.

**Ot-** **(G)** *pertaining to ear:* otorrhea, discharge from ear.

**Ovar-** **(G)** *pertaining to ovary:* ovariorrhexis, rupture of an ovary.

**Path-** **(G)** *pertaining to disease:* pathology, science of disease.

**Ped-** **(G)** *pertaining to children:* pediatrician, child specialist.

**Ped-** **(L)** *pertaining to feet:* pedograph, imprint of the foot.

**Pneum-** or **pneumon-** **(G)** *pertaining to lung (pneum–air):* pneumococcus, organism causing lobar pneumonia.

**Polio-** **(G)** *gray:* poliomyelitis, inflammation of gray substance of spinal cord.

**Proct-** **(G)** *pertaining to rectum:* proctectomy, surgical removal of rectum.

**Psych-** **(G)** *pertaining to mind:* psychiatry, treatment of mental disorders.

**Py-** **(G)** *pertaining to pus:* pyorrhea, discharge of pus.

**Pyel-** **(G)** *pertaining to pelvis:* pyelitis, inflammation of pelvis of kidney.

**Rach-** **(G)** *pertaining to spine:* rachicentesis, puncture into vertebral canal.

**Rhin-** **(G)** *pertaining to nose:* rhinology, knowledge concerning noses.

**Salping-** **(G)** *pertaining to tube:* salpingitis, inflammation of tube.

**Sapr-** **(G)** *pertaining to pus or decomposition:* saprophyte, vegetable organism living on dead or decaying vegetable matter.

**Septic-** **(L and G)** *pertaining to poison:* septicemia, poisoned condition of blood.

**Tox-** or **toxic-** **(G)** *pertaining to poison:* toxemia, poisoned condition of blood.

**Trache-** **(G)** *pertaining to the trachea:* tracheitis, inflammation of the trachea.

**Trich-** **(G)** *pertaining to the hair:* trichosis, any disease of the hair.

**Zoö-** **(G)** *pertaining to animal:* zoöblast, an animal cell.

## PREFIXES

**A-** or **An-** **(G)** *from, without:* asepsis, without infection.

**A-** or **Ab-** **(L)** *away, lack of:* abnormal, departing from the normal.

**Ad-** **(L)** *to, toward, near:* adrenal, near the kidney.

**Ambi-** **(L)** *both:* ambidextrous, referring to both hands.

**Ante-** **(L)** *before:* antenatal, occurring or having been formed before birth.

**Anti-** **(G)** *against:* antiseptic, against or preventing sepsis.

**Auto-** **(G)** *self:* auto-intoxication, poisoning by toxin generated in the body.

**Bi** or **Bin-** **(L)** *two:* binocular, pertaining to both eyes.

**Brady-** **(G)** *slow:* bradycardia, abnormal slowness of heartbeat.

**Circum-** **(L)** *around:* circumocular, around the eyes.

**Contra-** **(L)** *against, opposed:* contraindication, indication opposing usually indicated treatment.

**Counter-** **(L)** *against:* counterirritation, an irritation to relieve other irritation.

**Di-** **(L)** *two:* diphasic, occurring in two stages or phases.

**Dis-** **(L)** *apart:* disarticulation, taking joint apart.

**Dys-** **(G)** *pain or difficulty:* dyspepsia, impairment of digestion.

**Ecto-** **(G)** *outside:* ectoretina, outermost layer of retina.

**Em-** or **En-** **(G)** *in:* encapsulated, enclosed in a capsule.

**End-** **(G)** *within:* endothelium, layer of cells lining heart, blood and lymph vessels.

**Epi-** **(G)** *above or upon:* epidermis, outermost layer of skin.

**Erythro-** **(G)** *red:* erythrocyte, red blood cell.

**Eu-** **(G)** *well:* euphoria, well feeling, feeling of good health.

**Ex-** or **E-** **(L)** *out:* excretion, material thrown out of the body or the organ.

**Exo-** **(G)** *outside:* exocrine, excreting outwardly (opposite of endocrine).

**Extra-** **(G)** *outside:* extramural, situated or occurring outside a wall.

**Glyco-** **(G)** *sugar:* glycosuria, sugar in the urine.

**Hemi-** **(G)** *half:* heminephrectomy, excision of half the kidney.

**Hetero-** **(G)** *other (opposite of homo):* heterotransplant, using skin from a member of another species.

**Homo-** **(G)** *same:* homotransplant, skin grafting by using skin from a member of the same species.

**Hyper-** **(G)** *above, excess of:* hyperglycemia, excess of sugar in blood.

**Hypo-** **(G)** *under, deficiency of:* hypoglycemia, deficiency of sugar in blood.

**Im-** or **In-** **(L)** *in:* infiltration, accumulation in tissue of abnormal material.

**Im-** or **In** **(L)** *not:* immature, not mature.

**Infra-** **(L)** *below:* infraorbital, below the orbit.

**Inter-** **(L)** *between:* intermuscular, between the muscles.

**Intra-** **(L)** *within:* intramuscular, within the muscle.

**Macro-** **(G)** *large:* macroblast, abnormally large red cell.

**Meg-** or **Megal-** **(G)** *great:* megacolon, abnormally large colon.

**Mesa-** **(G)** *middle:* mesaortitis, inflammation of middle coat of the aorta.

**Meta-** **(G)** *beyond, over, change:* metastasis, change in site of a disease.

**Micro-** **(G)** *small:* microplasia, dwarfism.

**Mycet-** **(G)** *fungus:* mycetoma, tumor caused by a fungus.

**Olig-** **(G)** *little:* oligemia, deficiency in volume of blood.

**Para-** **(G)** *wrong, irregular, in the neighborhood of, around:* paradenitis, inflammation of tissue in the neighborhood of a gland.

**Per-** **(L)** *through, excessively:* percutaneous, through the skin.

**Peri-** **(G)** *around, immediately around* (in contradistinction to para): periapical, surrounding apex of root of tooth.

**Poly-** **(G)** *many:* polydactylism, many fingers, i.e., more than the usual five.

**Post-** **(L)** *after:* postpartum, after childbirth.

**Pre-** **(L)** *before:* prenatal, occurring before birth.

**Pro-** **(L and G)** *before:* prognosis, forecast as to result of disease.

**Pseud-** **(G)** *false:* pseudoangina, false angina.

**Retro-** **(L)** *backward:* retroversion, turned backward (usually, of uterus).

**Semi-** **(L)** *half:* semicoma, mild coma.

**Sub-** **(L)** *under:* subdiaphragmatic, under the diaphragm.

**Super-** **(L)** *above, excessively:* superacute, excessively acute.

**Supra-** **(L)** *above, upon:* suprarenal, above or upon the kidney.

**Sym-** or **Syn-** **(G)** *with, together:* symphysis, a growing together.

**Tachy-** **(G)** *fast:* tachycardia, fast-beating heart.

**Trans-** **(L)** *across:* transplant, transfer tissue from one place to another.

**Tri-** **(L and G)** *three:* trigastric, having three bellies (muscle).

**Uni-** **(L)** *one:* unilateral, affecting one side.

## SUFFIXES

**-algia** **(G)** *pain:* cardialgia, pain in the heart.

**-asis** or **-osis** **(G)** *affected with:* leukocytosis, excess number of leukocytes.

**-asthenia** **(G)** *weakness:* neurasthenia, nervous weakness.

**-blast** **(G)** *germ:* myeloblast, bone-marrow cell.

**-cele** **(G)** *tumor, hernia:* enterocele, any hernia of intestine.

**-clysis** **(G)** *injection:* hypodermoclysis, injection under the skin.

**-coccus** **(G)** *round bacterium:* pneumococcus, bacteria of pneumonia.

**-cyte (G)** *cell:* leukocyte, white cell.

**-ectasis (G)** *dilation, stretching:* angiectasis, dilatation of a blood vessel. This is really the same ending as *asis* or *osis,* and comes from the Greek, *ekt* or *ect.*

**-ectomy (G)** *excision:* adenectomy, excision of adenoids.

**-emia (G)** *blood:* glycemia, sugar in blood.

**-esthesia (G)** *(noun) relating to sensation:* anesthesia, absence of feeling.

**-genic (G)** *producing:* pyogenic, producing pus.

**-iatrics (G)** *pertaining to a physician or the practice of healing* (medicine): pediatrics, science of medicine for children.

**-itis (G)** *inflammation:* tonsillitis, inflammation of tonsils.

**-logy (G)** *science of:* pathology, science of disease.

**-lysis (G)** *losing, flowing, dissolution:* autolysis, dissolution of tissue cells.

**-malacia (G)** *softening:* osteomalacia, softening of bone.

**-oma (G)** *tumor:* myoma, tumor made up of muscle elements.

**-osis (-asis) (G)** *being affected with:* atherosis, arteriosclerosis.

**-(o)stomy (G)** *creation of an opening:* gastrostomy, creation of an artificial gastric fistula.

**-(o)tomy (G)** *cutting into:* laparotomy, surgical incision into the abdomen.

**-pathy (G)** *disease:* myopathy, disease of a muscle.

**-penia (G)** *lack of:* leukopenia, lack of white blood cells.

**-pexy (G)** *to fix:* proctopexy, fixation of rectum by suture.

**-phagia (G)** *eating:* polyphagia, excessive eating.

**-phasia (G)** *speech:* aphasia, loss of power of speech.

**-phobia (G)** *fear:* hydrophobia, fear of water.

**-plasty (G)** *molding:* gastroplasty, molding or re-forming stomach.

**-poiesis (G)** *making, forming:* hematopoiesis, forming blood.

**-pnea (G)** *air or breathing:* dyspnea, difficult breathing.

**-ptosis (G)** *falling:* enteroptosis, falling of intestine.

**-rhythmia (G)** *rhythm:* arrhythmia, variation from normal rhythm of heart.

**-rrhagia (G)** *flowing or bursting forth:* otorrhagia, hemorrhage from ear.

**-rrhaphy (G)** *suture of:* enterorrhaphy, act of sewing up gap in intestine.

**-rrhea (G)** *discharge:* otorrhea, discharge from ear.

**-rrhexis (G)** *rupture:* cardiorrhexis, rupture of heart.

**-sthen (ia) (ic) (G)** *pertaining to strength:* asthenia. loss of strength.

**-taxia** or **-taxis (G)** *order, arrangement of:* ataxia, failure of muscular coordination.

**-trophia** or **-trophy (G)** *nourishment:* atrophy, wasting, or diminution.

**-ultation (G)** *act of:* auscultation, listening for sound in body.

**-uria (G)** *to do with urine:* polyuria, excessive secretion of urine.

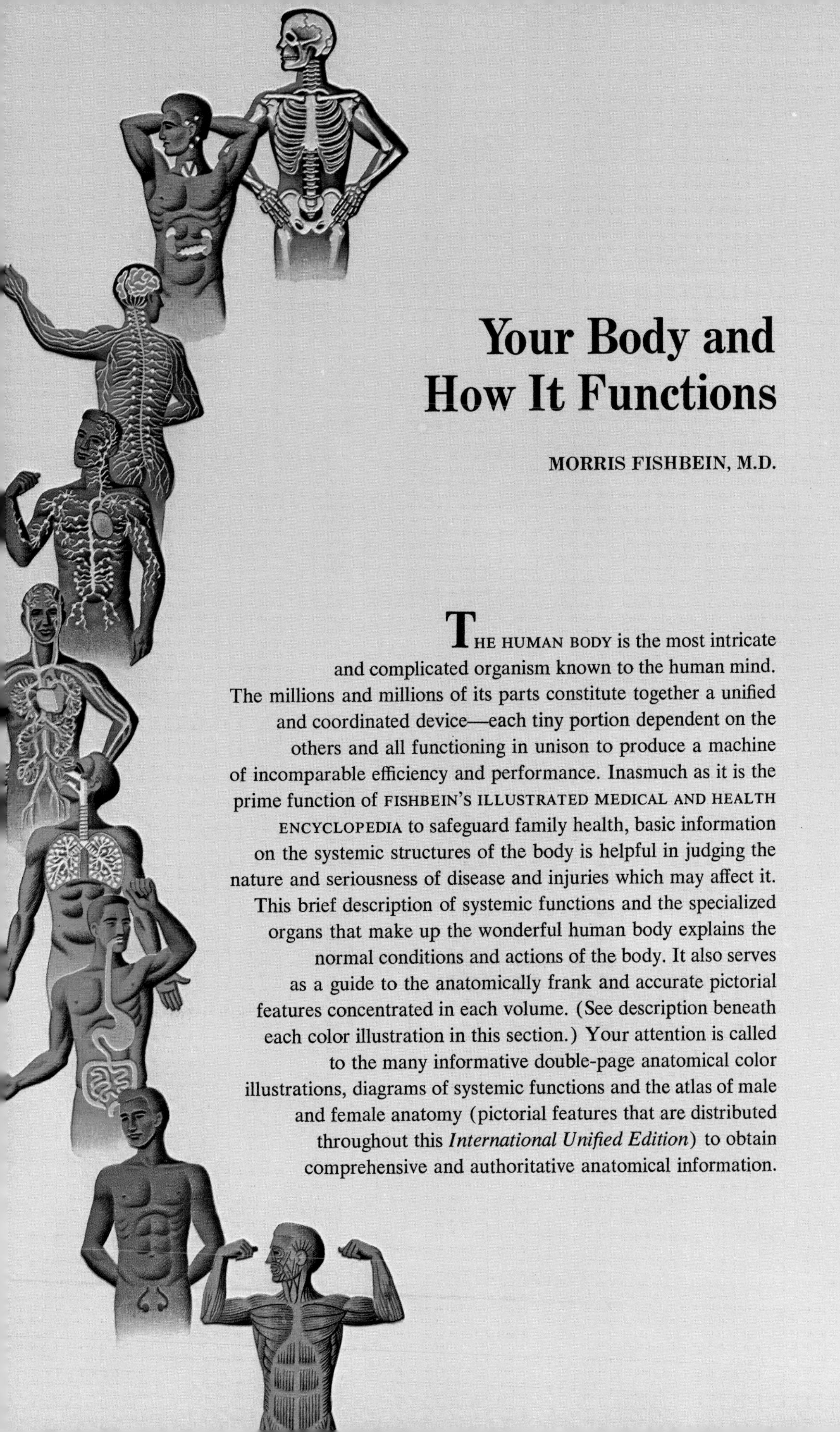

# Your Body and How It Functions

MORRIS FISHBEIN, M.D.

THE HUMAN BODY is the most intricate and complicated organism known to the human mind. The millions and millions of its parts constitute together a unified and coordinated device—each tiny portion dependent on the others and all functioning in unison to produce a machine of incomparable efficiency and performance. Inasmuch as it is the prime function of FISHBEIN'S ILLUSTRATED MEDICAL AND HEALTH ENCYCLOPEDIA to safeguard family health, basic information on the systemic structures of the body is helpful in judging the nature and seriousness of disease and injuries which may affect it. This brief description of systemic functions and the specialized organs that make up the wonderful human body explains the normal conditions and actions of the body. It also serves as a guide to the anatomically frank and accurate pictorial features concentrated in each volume. (See description beneath each color illustration in this section.) Your attention is called to the many informative double-page anatomical color illustrations, diagrams of systemic functions and the atlas of male and female anatomy (pictorial features that are distributed throughout this *International Unified Edition*) to obtain comprehensive and authoritative anatomical information.

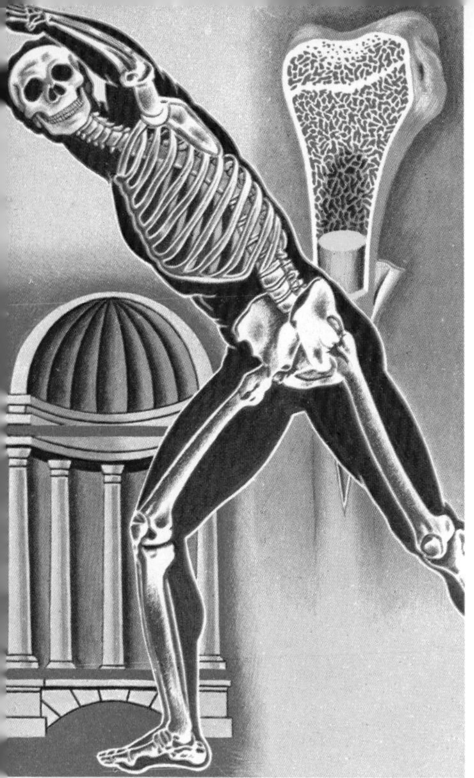

▲ An engineering marvel within you. The bones of your body must support a *growing* structure and protect its vital organs. See the **SKELETAL SYSTEM** anatomical illustrations in volume 20.

▼ More than 600 bundles consisting of billions of fine fibers make up the voluntary and involuntary muscles scattered throughout your body. See the **MUSCULAR SYSTEM** anatomical illustrations in volume 16.

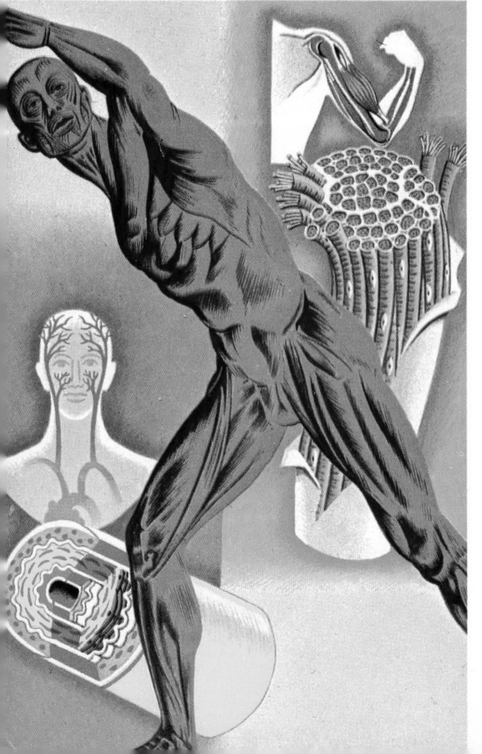

## The Bones

The bones of the human body, securely attached together by ligaments, form the skeleton or framework of the body. The body tissues, organs, and systems are located either inside the cavities formed by the skeleton or around it. The skeleton is the framework that holds everything in place. Also it is a source of attachment for many of the organs.

The skeleton or bony framework of the body accomplishes the following: (1) helps give shape to the body; (2) holds the body in an erect position; (3) forms cavities to hold and protect vital organs; and (4) provides strength, firmness, and leverage.

The bones of the skeleton may be classified into three groups, including: (1) the bones of the head or skull; (2) the bones of the body or trunk; (3) the bones of the limbs, including both arms and legs.

Joints connect the ends of two or more bones where they come together. The bones forming a joint are held together by strong white bands of connective tissue called ligaments.

Some joints are fixed or immovable, such as those of the skull of an adult. Other joints are movable although the extent of movement permitted is not always the same. In the case of the backbone and wrist, movement is limited. The elbow and knee joints allow free bending and extending of the parts. The hip and shoulder joints, called ball-and-socket joints, allow free movement in every direction.

Sometimes the ligaments binding the bones together are injured by being torn or overstretched when bones are thrown out of place at a joint.

## The Muscles

The bony framework of the body is covered by muscles. They are attached to the bones. The cavities of the body are enclosed by muscles which protect the organs in the cavities.

The muscles produce movement and help in supporting the skeleton. Finally, the muscles produce a large part of the body bulk. They are important to the health of the body in many ways.

Muscles are voluntary and involuntary. The voluntary muscles, such as those used in walking or lifting, are under conscious control. The involuntary muscles, such as the heart and those involved in breathing and digestion, are beyond our control.

Tendons are the bands by which muscles are attached to bones. They are strong bands of white glistening cords formed by the extension of sheaths covering the muscle fibers. Movement of the body is produced when muscles contract or shorten. The tendons of muscles are attached to the bone; thus when the muscle grows shorter, the bones are pulled together to make the movement.

### The Nervous System

The body is provided with a sturdy frame in the form of a bony skeleton and hundreds of muscles are arranged in and around the body framework to provide a means of movement. This entire mechanism would be useless without some centralized means of control and coordination.

The human body depends upon its nervous system to control, regulate, and stimulate the many parts of the human machine.

The nervous system of the body is divided into two parts: the cerebrospinal system and the autonomic system. The cerebrospinal system is composed of the brain and the spinal nerves. It is the basis of consciousness and coordinates the responses and movements made due to sensations. Sensations pass from small nerves to the uttermost parts of the body up to the brain; from the brain impulses go back to muscles and other tissues of the body. The autonomic system supplies the involuntary muscles just discussed.

### The Digestive System

Growth, repair, heat, and energy materials are essential to the body. The food we eat supplies these important materials; however, food cannot be used for growth, repair, heat, and energy until certain changes occur. The digestive system along with the circulatory and respiratory systems makes it possible for the body to use the food we eat to maintain life.

Food is digested in the alimentary canal—that is, the mouth, esophagus, stomach, and small and large intestine. It is first chewed and mixed with saliva. Then it is swallowed and passes down the esophagus or food pipe to the stomach. The movement of food in the alimentary canal is accomplished through the action of muscle fibers in the wall of the canal.

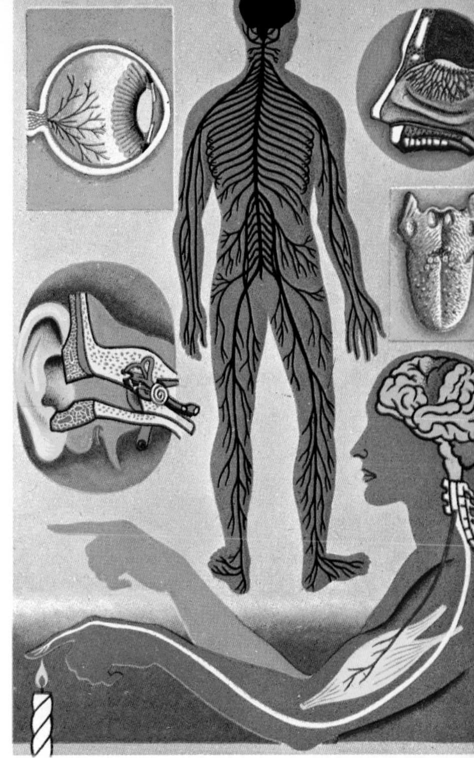

▲ The nerves function just like a radar and computer network! They collect, sort and file data and make it instantly available for *automatic* action. See the **NERVOUS SYSTEM** anatomical illustrations in volume 2.

▼ Your digestive system may be compared with a chemical engine that selects and refines its own fuel to provide energy. See the **DIGESTIVE SYSTEM** anatomical illustrations in volume 7.

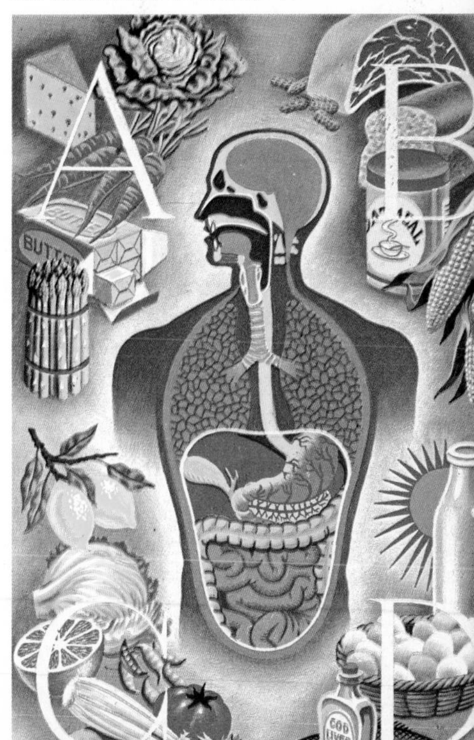

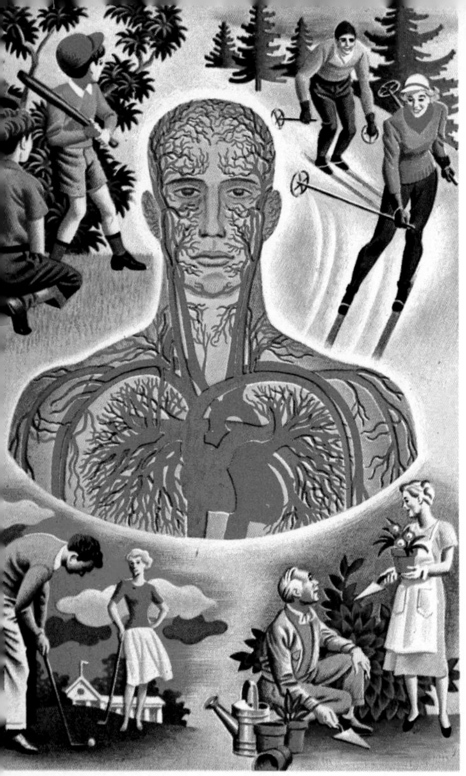

▲ Your heart is a bundle of muscles about the size of a fist. An understanding of its normal functions can help you achieve long, active, and vigorous life. See the **CIRCULATORY SYSTEM** anatomical illustrations in volume 5.

▼ Various glands produce the hormones that are masters of your body, controlling its growth and regulating its activities to satisfy the body needs. See the **ENDOCRINE SYSTEM** anatomical illustrations in volume 8.

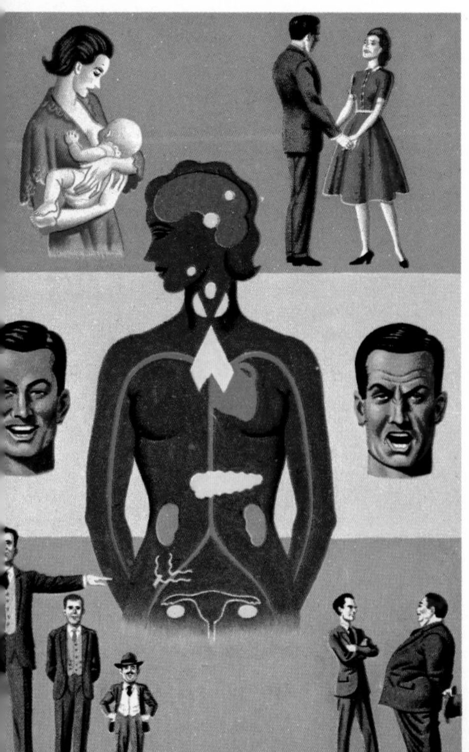

Part of the food which reaches the stomach is digested by the action of the gastric, or digestive, juices. The gastric juices are secreted by glands which become active when food enters the stomach.

The food passes from the stomach into the small intestine, where the process of digestion is continued and completed. In the small intestine the digested food is absorbed into the blood through the thin walls of the blood vessels. The indigestible parts of the food pass from the small intestine to the large intestine and then out of the body.

### The Circulatory System

After the food is digested, it is carried to all parts of the body where it is used to build new tissue. The circulatory system is the means by which the food is transported.

The blood is circulated throughout the body through blood vessels: arteries, veins, and capillaries. As it circulates throughout the body the blood performs a number of important duties. First, it carries food, fuels, and oxygen to all parts of the body. Second, it collects waste materials and returns them to be eliminated from the body. Third, it helps in regulating the body temperature.

The blood is composed largely of a liquid called plasma. Both red and white corpuscles are found in the plasma. The red cells carry oxygen to all parts of the body. The white cells, larger than the red cells and much less numerous, have the ability to pass through thin walls of the capillaries into the tissue. They form a protection against germs that enter the body by collecting in large numbers wherever germs are found.

### The Heart

The pumping action of the heart ceases only with death. Day and night, year after year, it continues to work in pumping the blood throughout the body. It can rest only by pumping more slowly or less powerfully.

The heart is a hollow, pear-shaped muscular organ located just slightly to the left of the midline of the body in the chest cavity. It can be located easily by the sound of the heartbeat or the feeling of its contraction through the skin and muscle that lie over it.

# SITES OF PAIN

## Their possible significance

Pain is nature's warning sign of wrong functioning or disease. It is a valuable indicator in the detection of ailing parts. Persistent, localized pain should never be ignored. It calls for thorough medical investigation.

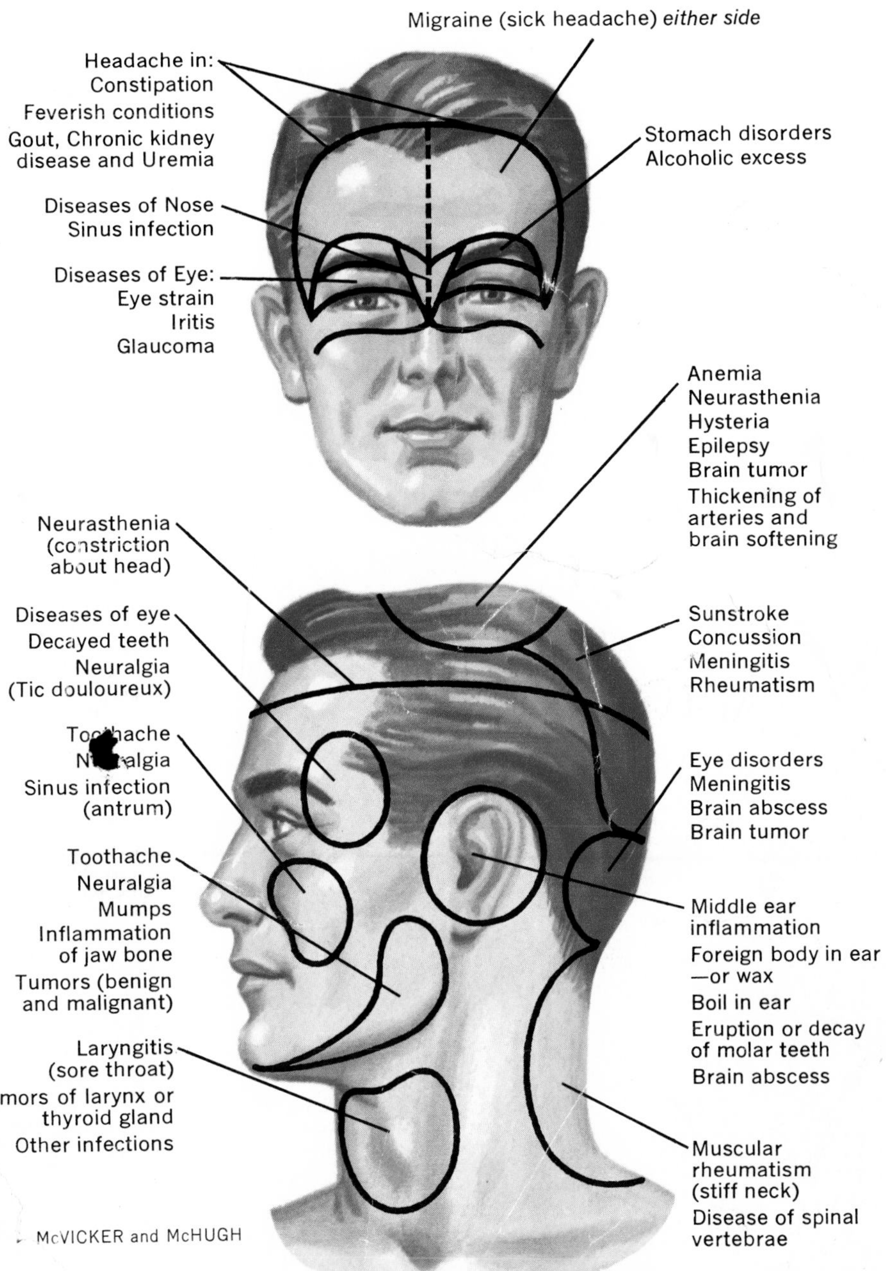


**HEADACHES AND PAINS OF FACE AND NECK**

## of Pain

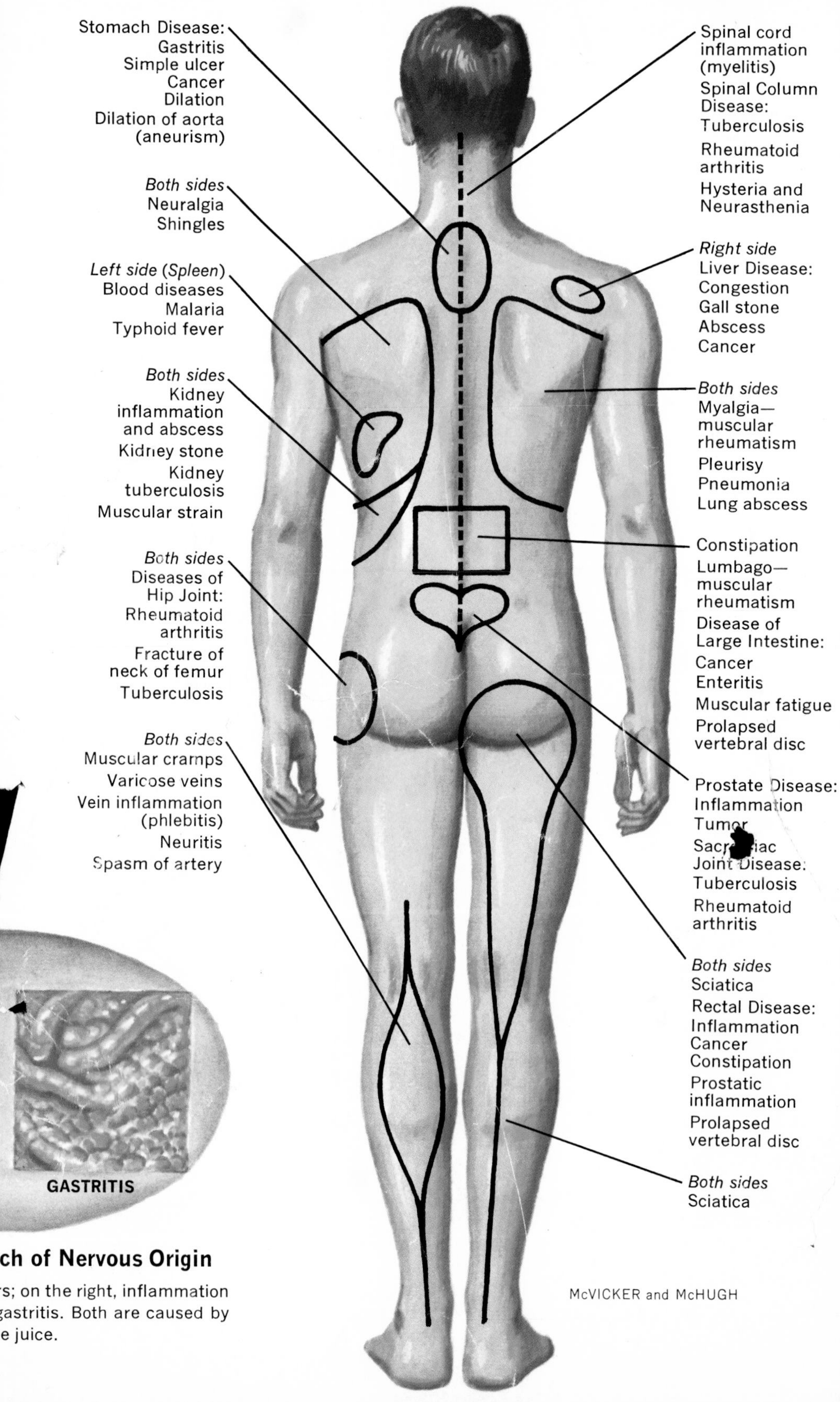


## ach of Nervous Origin

ers; on the right, inflammation -gastritis. Both are caused by ve juice.

At birth the heart beats about 130 times a minute, at six years it beats 100 times a minute, at ten years about 90, and at fifteen years about 85. The approximate normal heart rate among adults ranges from 65 to 80 beats per minute. During a lifetime the heart beats 2,500,000,000 times and pumps a total of nearly 15,000,000 gallons.

The impulse which causes the heart to contract develops in some nerve tissue which is called the pacemaker of the heart. An attempt to measure this impulse indicates that its energy is the equivalent of one-thousandth of a volt.

The blood from all parts of the body empties into the heart through large veins. Then it is sent through the lungs, where it acquires a new supply of oxygen. The blood then returns to the heart from the lungs. When the heart muscle contracts, the blood is forced out of the heart, then goes by way of the large arteries and capillaries to the farthest extremes of the body.

The heart moves a total of five hundred gallons of blood a day. Since there are about six quarts of blood in the whole body, the heart moves the same fluid, slightly modified chemically as it travels about, over and over again.

### Arteries, Veins, and Capillaries

The blood vessels which carry the bright red oxygenated blood away from the heart are called arteries. The large arteries, which receive the blood directly from the heart, branch repeatedly until every part of the body is served by one or more of them.

The blood returns from all parts of the body to the heart through veins. There are many more veins than arteries throughout the body. The veins gradually unite to form larger veins as they approach the heart.

When the blood is sent out over the body through the arteries it passes into the capillaries in which the arteries end. The capillaries are tiny hairlike blood vessels forming a network throughout the body. The tissue is so well supplied with capillaries that even a pinprick is likely to break some of them and result in the appearance of a few drops of blood.

When an artery, vein, or capillary is broken or cut, blood flows from the broken vessels. Usually

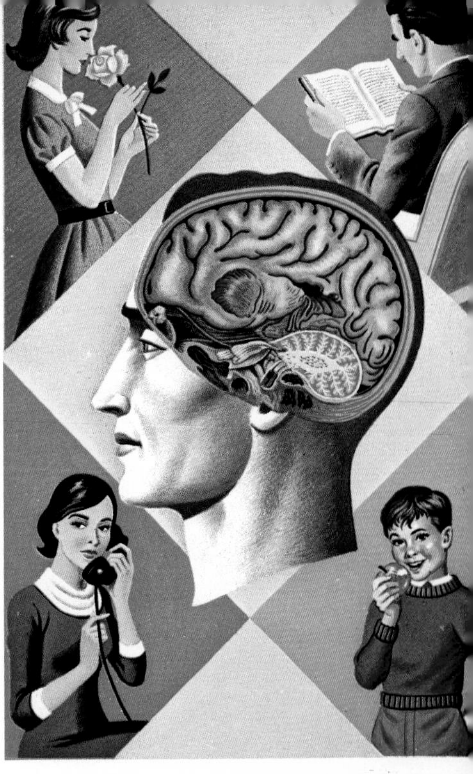

▲ You perceive the world around you through the senses of *sight, sound, taste,* and *smell.* All the organs of these senses are linked to the nervous system. See the **SPECIAL SENSE ORGANS** anatomical illustrations in volume 21.

▼ These vital fluids circulate in a vast network of veins, arteries, and capillaries to transport food to the cells and protect them against bacterial invasion. See the **BLOOD AND LYMPHATIC SYSTEM** anatomical illustrations in volume 4.

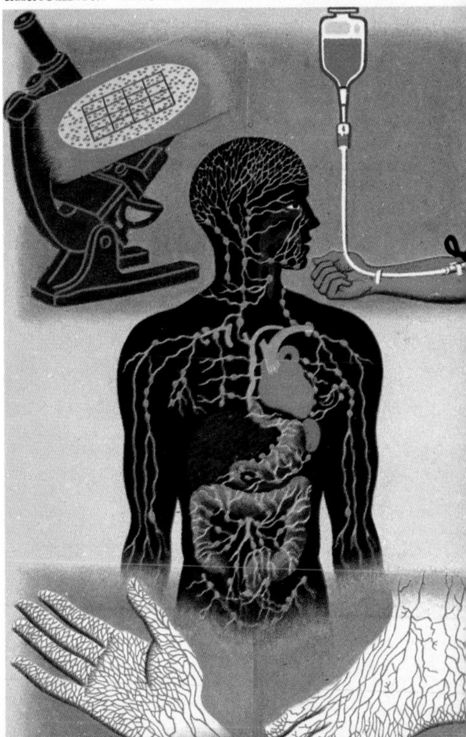

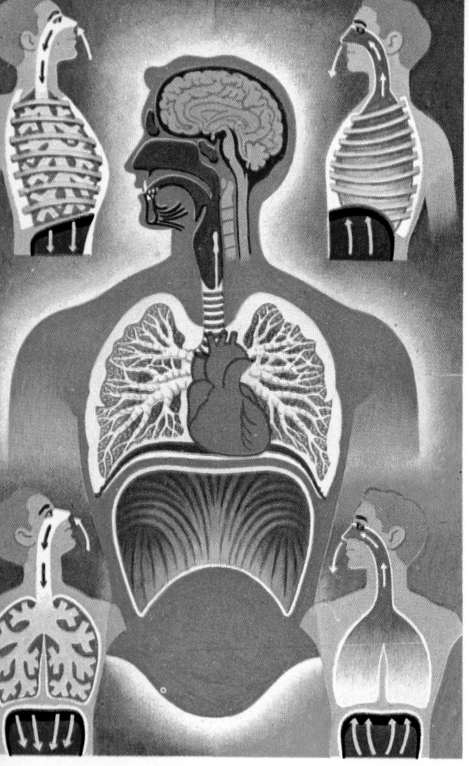

▲ The lungs, diaphragm, and respiratory centers are part of a living bellows—governing the process of combining oxygen and food substances to produce energy. See the **RESPIRATORY SYSTEM** anatomical illustrations in volume 19.

▼ Conception, development, birth . . . creating *new* life is the most miraculous act of living. See the **BIRTH, DEVELOPMENT AND GROWTH** anatomical illustrations in volume 3.

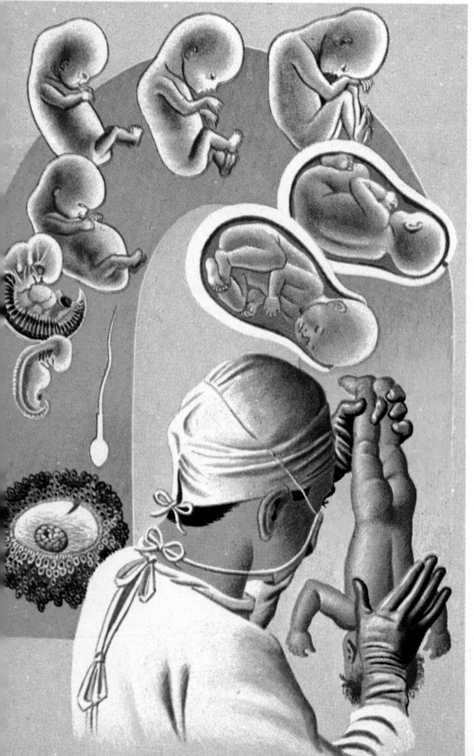

the blood flow from the broken blood vessels is stopped by the formation of a clot in the end of the broken vessels. Bleeding from a large artery is extremely serious. The blood from a severed artery comes in spurts. There is a smooth flow of blood from veins.

### The Lymphatics

A large part of the human body is composed of connective tissue. Within this connective tissue are the lymph cells and the walls of the lymph vessels. The connective tissue is concerned in the formation of blood and blood vessels and also in the formation of lymph vessels.

Through the lymph vessels the white blood cells, which pick up waste material from the body, travel carrying the remains of dead tissue and foreign bodies. The lymph capillaries correspond also to the blood capillaries, the tiniest vessels which form the connection between the arterial and venous blood systems.

The lymph vessels take up fluid from the tissue spaces. Along the lymph vessels are lymph glands. Every lymph vessel passes through a lymph gland somewhere. These glands are spongelike filters. Many blood vessels enter all around their surface but only one or two blood vessels leave. The lymph oozes through the sponge material composed largely of white blood cells which develop and pass into the blood. Movement of the lymph is facilitated by muscle action. Indeed every movement of the body helps to stimulate the lymphatic circulation.

### The Respiratory System

Breathing or respiration is the means by which the body is supplied with air containing oxygen. The organs of breathing or respiration include the nose, mouth, throat, epiglottis, trachea or windpipe, bronchial tubes, and lungs.

The breathing of air into the lungs is called inspiration. This is caused by an enlargement of the chest cavity through the action of muscles pulling the ribs upward and outward. At the same time the large domeshaped diaphragm muscle which separates the chest cavity from the abdominal cavity pushes downward to help enlarge the chest cavity.

Breathing out, or expiration is caused by the muscles forcing a decrease in the size of the chest cavity.

The rate of breathing or respiration varies with the individual. Adults breathe approximately fifteen to eighteen times per minute although this number may vary.

Respiration is under the control of the nervous system just like other body functions vital to life. The breathing center of the nervous system which controls respiration is located in the brain.

When the air is drawn in through the nose or mouth, it passes into the windpipe from the throat. The top of the windpipe is protected by a little flap called the epiglottis. When one swallows, the epiglottis closes over the top of the windpipe to keep food or liquids from entering the windpipe.

The air passes down the windpipe into the bronchial tubes. The bronchial tubes end in the air sacs. The walls of the air sacs contain a network of capillaries. As the blood goes through the capillaries, the oxygen from the air in the air sacs passes through the thin walls and is taken up by the red cells of the blood. Carbon dioxide in the blood passes through the capillaries into the lungs where it is expired.

## Skin

The skin of the human body is living tissue, not just an envelope to cover the surface and hold in the organs. The skin of a grown person weighs about six pounds. If spread flat it would cover sixteen to twenty square feet.

The skin on the palms of the hands, the soles of the feet, the shoulders, and the back of the neck is the thickest on the body. It varies from 2/100 to 16/100 of an inch in thickness. Like other living tissue of which the human body is composed, the skin tends to regulate its own condition fairly well.

The skin performs a number of important functions. It protects the body against invasion of bacteria, against harmful rays of the sun, and against loss of moisture. It also serves as the perceptive organ for the nervous system, perceiving pain, pressure, heat and cold. A further function performed by the skin, is the regulation of body temperature through the dilation and contraction of the many blood vessels contained in the skin.

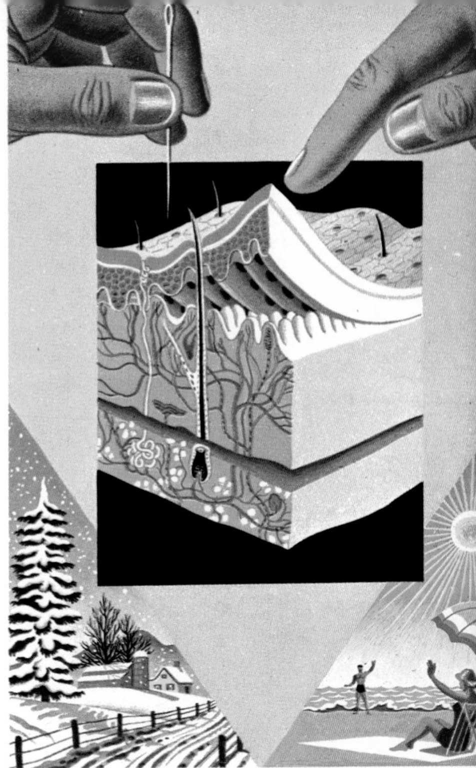

▲ Skin is living tissue to protect your body against bacterial invasion, perceive external conditions for the nerves and regulate body temperature. See the **SKIN AND HAIR** anatomical illustrations in volume 11.

▼ Pain is nature's warning sign of disease or malfunctions in the body . . . each site of pain has its specific significance. See the **SITES OF PAIN** anatomical illustrations in volume 1.

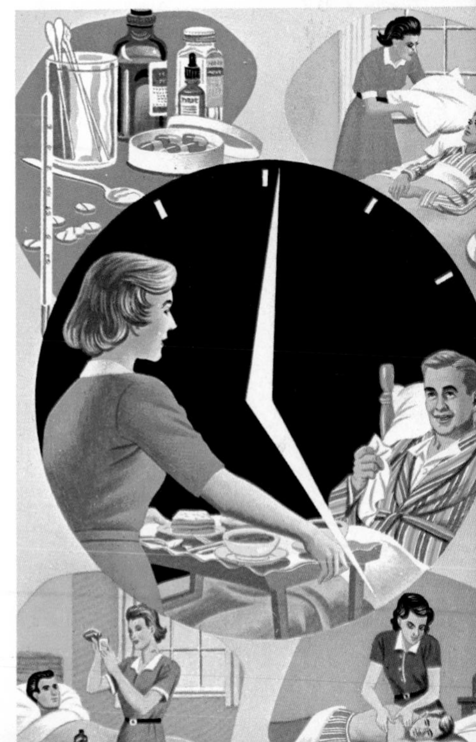

## Excretion

Most of what we eat and swallow is digested and absorbed from the intestines. When the blood has taken up an excess of protein from the intestine this excess must be eliminated.

In the skin the sweat glands aid to rid the body not only of some excess fluid but also of various substances which are dissolved in the fluid.

The cells that line the intestines not only take up useful material but also eliminate waste material. The greater part of elimination of substances from the blood is accomplished by the two kidneys. They throw out in the form of urine considerable amounts of substances which are unnecessary to the body. From the kidneys the material passes down the ureters, into the urinary bladder. The capacity of the bladder is a little less than one pint but it may be distended to hold one and a half pints.

From the bladder the material passes through a tube called the urethra. Valves control the flow of excretion through this tube.

Thus excretion is carried on in the body through the bowel, solid waste material going out through the rectum and anus, fluid material through the kidneys, and additional fluid material through the sweat glands.

## The Glands

Within the body there is an interlocking chain of glands which produce hormones that regulate the functions of various organs and tissues. The glands which produce chemical substances that pass directly into the blood are the pituitary gland, the thyroid, the parathyroids, the pancreas, the suprarenal glands or adrenals, and the sex glands which include the ovaries of the woman and the testicles of the man. These internal secretions are essential to reproduction, to growth, to health, and to life.

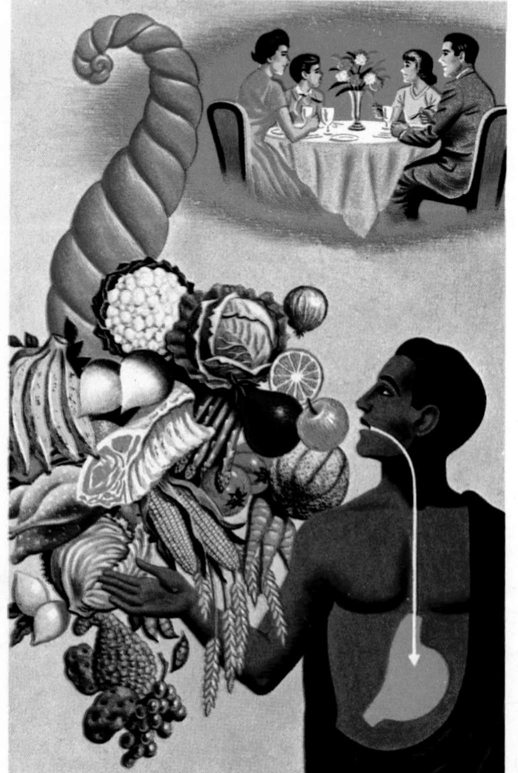

◀ Vitamins have special virtues. An understanding of nutrition helps maintain all body systems and keeps them functioning properly. See the special article, **Vitamins—The Cornerstones of Health,** in volume 22.

## Sites

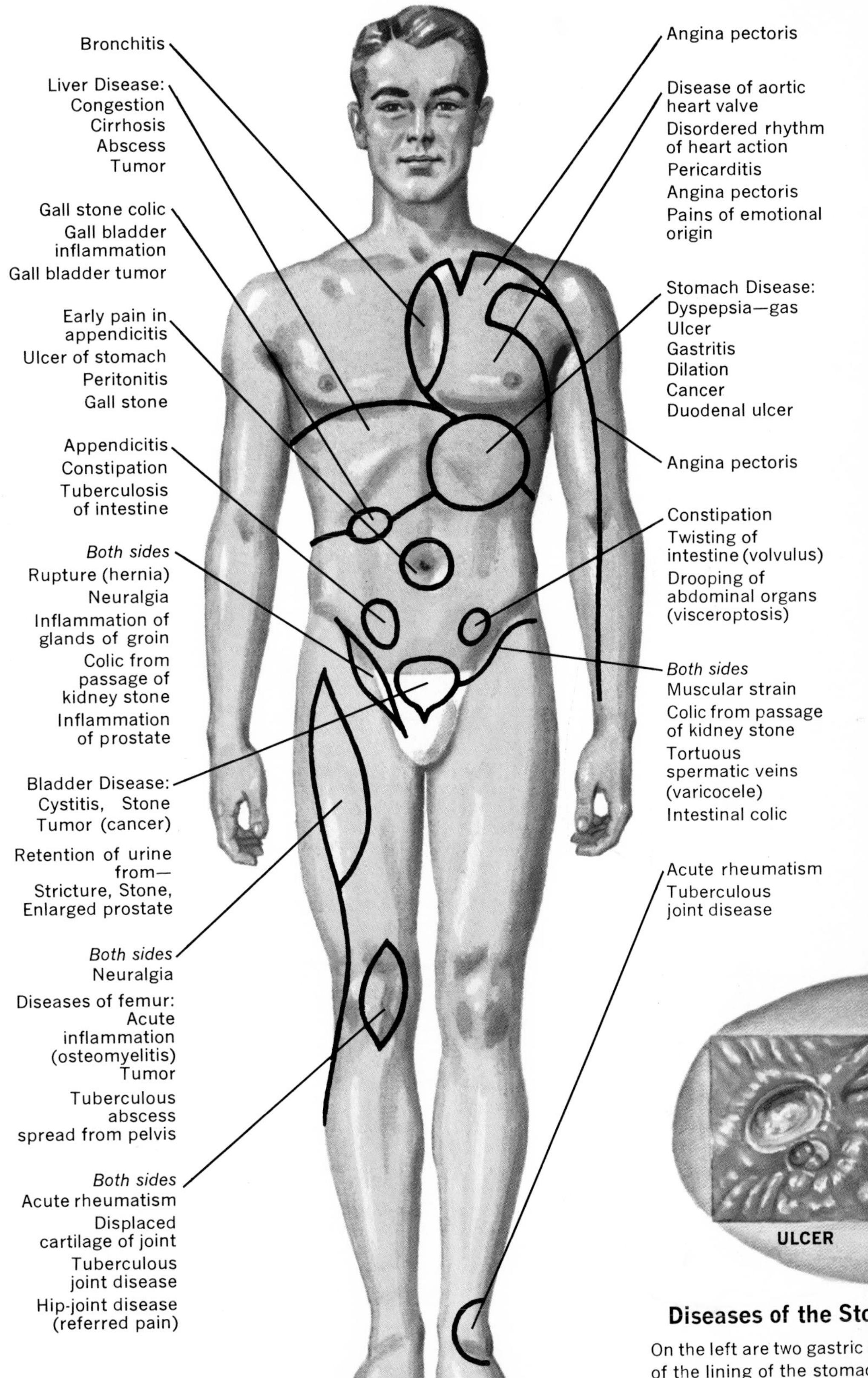


### Diseases of the Stor

On the left are two gastric ul
of the lining of the stomach
overproduction of acid dige

## Sites of Pain

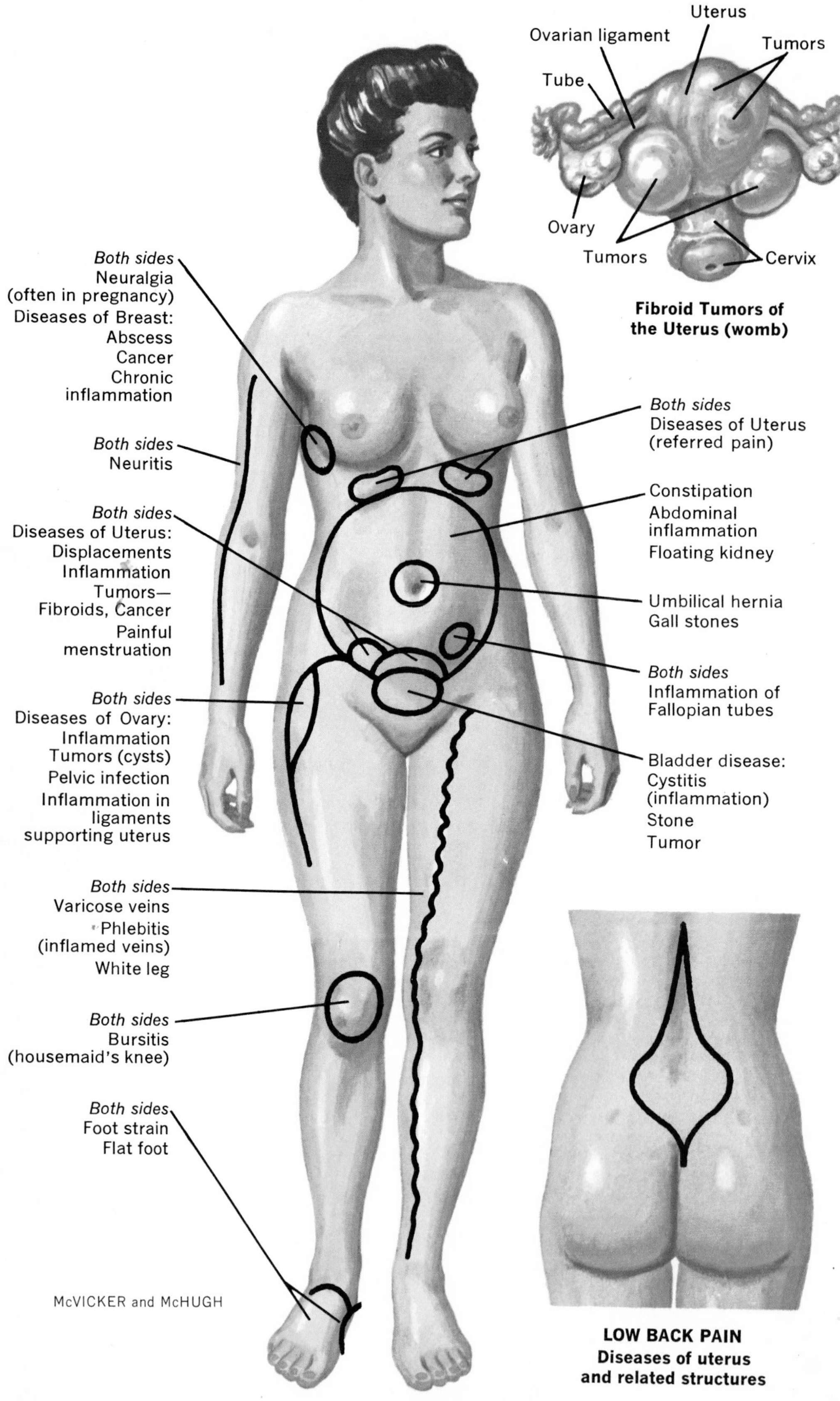


**LOW BACK PAIN**
**Diseases of uterus and related structures**

# A

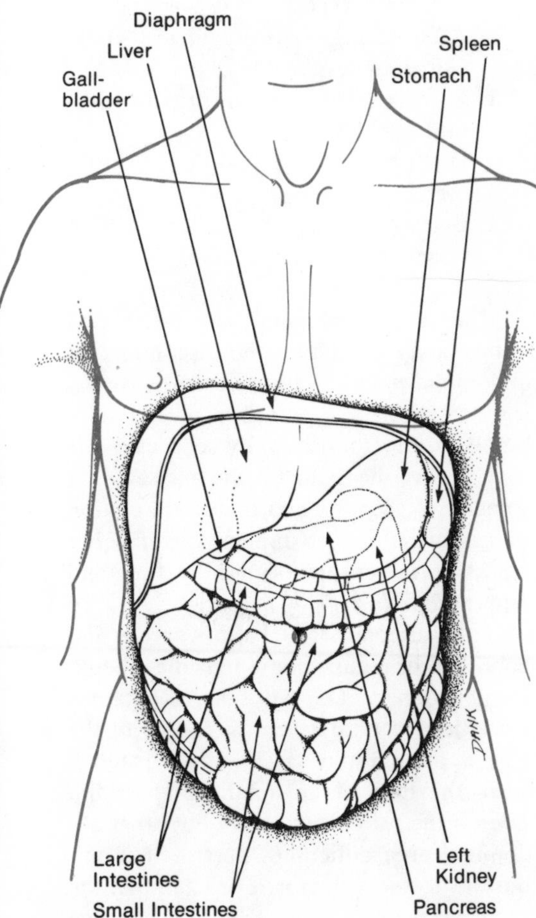


**Abdomen**—The organs of digestion, absorption and elimination are located in the abdomen. They are grouped together in a way that produces maximum efficiency in the various functions and interactions—as long as the organs themselves are free of disease or injury.

**ABASIA,** the inability to walk, caused by loss of coordination. Muscular spasms, spastic stiffening, or paralysis can cause this condition. *See* LEG; PARALYSIS.

**ABDOMEN,** the portion of the body between the lower part of the chest and the pelvis. This oval-shaped cavity is separated from the chest by the *diaphragm.* Heavy muscles protect the abdomen in the front and sides, and the spinal column with its muscles protects it in back. The abdomen is lined by a membrane, the *peritoneum.* The *stomach, large* and *small intestines, liver, spleen, pancreas, kidneys, appendix, gallbladder, urinary bladder,* major *blood vessels,* and *nerves* lie within the abdomen. Many people call this area by the common term *belly.*

The function of abdominal organs is the digestion of food, absorption of nutrients by the body, and elimination of indigestible substances and wastes. In the female, the sexual organs are also located within the abdomen, whereas the male sex organs lie adjacent to it.

The abdominal walls not only protect the organs but hold them in place so that they can function properly. *See also* ABDOMINAL PAIN.

**ABDOMINAL PAIN,** technically called *abdominalgia,* a pain or discomfort in the abdomen which signifies an abdominal disorder. Anyone suffering such pain should be cautious about treating it with-

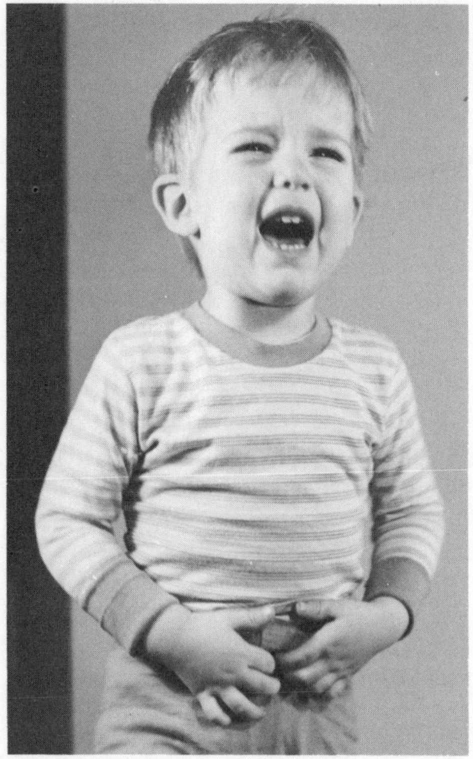

**Abdominal Pain**—It can be difficult to determine the cause of children's stomach aches. All they can tell you is that "it hurts." Perhaps this youngster ate unripe fruit or contaminated food. Or he may have been overly active too soon after a full meal. When pain persists or the child is feverish, a doctor should be consulted.

out a doctor's advice. Discomfort may be temporary, such as that caused simply by overeating; or it may be serious, resulting from an inflamed appendix, an infection, or a tumor.

Excessive eating, drinking, or smoking can cause abdominal pain. Anxiety, stress, fear, or emotional problems can lead to abdominal pain. If frequent or prolonged, these difficulties may bring about actual damage—for example, an ulcerated stomach.

The "stomach ache"—a general feeling of discomfort—usually disappears after a few hours. Recurrent or continuing pain, however, should have a doctor's attention.

Since so many different problems can cause abdominal pain, doctors ask many questions when they try to find a cause. Such questions include these:

1. Has the pain occurred before? If so, how often?
2. Does the pain remain in one part of the abdomen? If not, where else does it occur?
3. In which of the six areas of the abdomen does the pain occur: the pit of the stomach; around the navel; in one of the four quadrants (upper right, upper left, lower right, or lower left)?
4. After eating, is the pain the same, worse, or lessened?
5. Is there nausea or diarrhea in addition to the pain?
6. Describe the pain—dull, sharp, crampy, pressing?
7. Is the pain eased by walking, sitting down, lying on the back, lying on the side?

Mild occasional pain may be treated immediately at home. The discomfort of abdominal pain can be relieved by drinking hot strong tea or a cup of hot salty bouillon. Dry toast or salty soda crackers may lessen the pain or the nausea that sometimes accompanies the accumulation of gas or acid. The application of a hot water bottle or an electric heating pad may be helpful.

If the discomfort or pain is severe and continues or recurs, home remedies should be abandoned. Do not take a laxative, since this may not reach the source of the pain at all and may cause serious trouble, as in the case of an inflamed appendix. Even if the pain is not severe but other abdominal area difficulties persist, it is important to see a doctor. For example, the early stages of cancer do not produce much pain, but other symptoms, including loss of weight or bloody urine or feces, may occur. Diagnosing abdominal pain is difficult and complex enough for a physician. Therefore, you should not try to diagnose and treat such pain yourself.

*Upper Abdominal Pain.* Sharp or acute pain, vomiting, and diarrhea sometimes indicate food poisoning. Medication should not be taken unless prescribed by a doctor.

Recurring pain and mild or severe discomfort in the upper abdomen, accompanied by nausea, indigestion, and intolerance to fatty foods, may mean that stones have formed in the gallbladder. Gallstones are formed when certain chemicals, found in bile, begin to harden and settle in the gallbladder. If one of these stones enters a gallbladder duct, severe cramping or colic may be felt as it passes through the passage.

Sharp pain anywhere in the abdomen may be caused by poisoning, an overdose of strong drugs, or deficiency disorders, such as *pernicious anemia* or *sprue*. Certain infectious diseases, such as *pneumonia* or *infectious mononucleosis,* may include among their symptoms severe abdominal pain.

Pain accompanied by *jaundice*—a yellowing of the skin and eyes—may follow the complications of either a gallbladder or a liver disorder. The pain itself may be mild or even absent. When pressure applied to the right upper sector of the abdomen causes pain, the condition may be hepatitis or another liver ailment.

An ulcer—an open sore anywhere in the upper abdomen—may cause a burning pain. The sore may be on the lining of the stomach itself or in the connecting *duodenum,* the first portion of the small intestine. Someone with an ulcer may feel pain two or three hours after a meal, or he may be awakened in the middle of the night. He may vomit, and blood may appear in his vomit or feces. If the ulcer perforates through the wall of the organ —usually without warning—agonizing pain occurs in the upper abdomen. Such a situation is serious and requires immediate medical attention.

Pain in the upper abdomen may be caused by *pleurisy,* an inflammation of the membrane that covers the lungs and surfaces of the chest cavity. This becomes worse when the sufferer coughs or breathes deeply. The pain of pleurisy is one of many pains that can occur in the abdomen although the cause lies elsewhere in the body.

*Lower Abdominal Pain.* Inflammation of the appendix, or *appendicitis,* is the most common cause of lower abdominal pain. It may begin in the center of the abdomen, then usually—though not always—move to the lower right sector. In addition to pain, the victim may suffer nausea and fever. In children, the fever will be higher than in adults. The pain may be mild, but will become more intense if pressure is applied. If you suspect appendicitis, never give a laxative; do not eat or drink; do not give any pain-killer or other medication; and do not use a hot water bottle. The only safe home treatment is to apply an ice pack until a doctor can examine the patient. If the pain stops suddenly, this may mean that the appendix has burst, creating a far more serious condition than the original appendicitis itself.

Constipation can cause pain and a feeling of fullness in the rectal area. Constipation may be caused by faulty diet, emotional upset, or weakness of the abdominal muscles. It may also be a symptom of a more serious condition. If it persists, a doctor should be consulted.

Women may suffer lower abdominal pain during menstruation. They may experience menstrual cramps not only in the lower abdomen but also in the back or down the legs. If the pain occurs midway between menstrual periods, it can range from mild to severe. Such pain, which may be confused with appendicitis, is caused by the normal process of the *ovum*—egg—leaving the ovary and beginning its passage to the uterus, a monthly occurrence called *ovulation.*

Other causes of lower abdominal pain in women include disorders of the lining of the uterus; infection of the Fallopian tubes; and rarely, *ectopic pregnancy*—pregnancy occurring in the Fallopian tubes instead of in the uterus.

An obstruction in the large intestine causes cramplike pain, with constipation, vomiting, and abdominal tenderness. *Intussusception,* a condition in which a part of the bowel telescopes into itself, sometimes appears in young children. Blocking also may be caused by *adhesions,* tumors, or ruptures in the abdominal wall.

Many other conditions may cause abdominal pain or discomfort. *See also* CANCER; DIGESTION; DIGESTIVE SYSTEM; FOOD POISONING; GASTROENTERITIS; PEPTIC ULCER *and* **medigraphs** APPENDICITIS; BOTULISM; CIRRHOSIS OF THE LIVER; GALLSTONES; GASTRITIS; ILEITIS; KIDNEY STONES; LEAD POISONING; PANCREATIC CANCER; PANCREATITIS; STOMACH CANCER; ULCERATIVE COLITIS; ULCERS OF THE DIGESTIVE TRACT.

▶ Digestive Diseases, *Common Symptoms,* 918. Infectious Diseases, *Typhoid Fever,* 1737; *Dysentery,* 1739.

RESEARCH REPORT

COMMON "GAS PAIN" COMPLAINT DUE TO FAULTY MOTILITY, NOT EXCESS AMOUNT

Objective measurements of abdominal gas volume indicate that patients who complain of bloating and cramps because of "too much gas" are actually suffering from a condition in which a normal amount of intestinal gas has a tendency to move too slowly and reflux back into the stomach. Challenging the accepted notion that excessive gas is a cause of gastrointestinal discomfort, a UNIVERSITY OF MINNESOTA research team had previously determined the volume and composition of human intestinal gas. They used this information to study a group of 18 patients with chronic complaints of excess gas.

Employing a method known as *washout technique,* which involved infusing an inert gas mixture into the intestine of the patients and of a group of normal control subjects, the researchers then collected and analyzed the endogenous gas that was displaced.

Results indicated that there was no significant difference in intestinal gas volume between both sets of subjects, nor was there a difference in chemical composition or the accumulation rate of intestinal gas.

The complaints of discomfort were valid nonetheless: the gas infused into the patients did produce more unpleasant symptoms than in normal subjects and it had a greater tendency to move back into the stomach. In addition, in all the patients for whom the gas infusions had to be terminated because they caused so much pain, the transit time of the gas through the intestine took about *twice* as long (40 minutes) as it did for the controls (22 minutes). Thus, even though the common complaint of "too much gas" is an inaccurate description of the cause of discomfort, a reduction in the gas volume might be a countermeasure for the sluggishness with which the gas moves. NIH116

**ABDOMINAL SUPPORTS,** devices which help to hold abdominal muscles or organs in place. Muscles may become weakened by disease or may become nonsupportive in old age. Abdominal supports may help to correct such malfunctions; but they should not be used unless prescribed by a doctor who has examined the offending condition.

An abdominal support may be prescribed to relieve backache. The support takes weight and stress off the spinal column, relieving the pain, and helps the individual maintain better posture.

The added pressure on—and resulting sagging of—the abdominal wall during pregnancy can be relieved by a special support.

One of the many complications of overweight is a weakened, strained, and sagging abdominal wall. A support may be advised; but of course, the only long-term

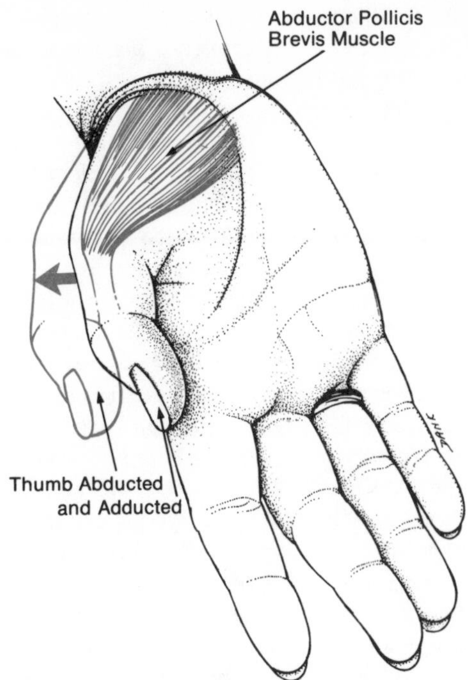


**Abductor**—The abductor muscle of the thumb enables it to draw away from the hand. This is an essential action in the hundreds of hand movements a person makes every day. The adductor muscle draws the thumb back to the hand.

relief for this abdominal problem is to lose the excess weight.

A support may be needed temporarily after certain types of abdominal operations. It also may be used in cases of hernia, although here too, a support is not a cure but only a method giving relief. *See also* HERNIA; TRUSS *and* **medigraph** INGUINAL HERNIA.

**ABDUCTOR,** a muscle that draws a part away (abducts) from the body or an extremity. An abductor muscle may be tiny (as in the fingers and toes) or large and powerful (as in the thighs). The principal abductor muscles include the *abductor digiti minimi* (which abducts the little finger in the hand and the little toe in the foot); the *abductor hallucis* (which abducts and flexes the big toe); the *abductor pollicis brevis* (which abducts the thumb); the *abductor pollicis longus* (which abducts and extends the thumb); the *deltoideus* (which abducts, flexes, and extends the arm); the *gluteus maximus* or buttock (which extends, abducts, and rotates the thigh outward); the *extensor carpi radialis brevis* and *extensor carpi radialis longus* (which extend and abduct the wrist joint); and the *interossei dorsales* (which abduct and flex the toes).

An *adductor* muscle is one that draws a part toward the body. *See also* ADDUCTOR; MUSCLES *and* **medigraph** SPRAINS AND STRAINS.

**ABERRATION,** a deviation from normality, whether in development or behavior. A *chromosomal aberration* is a deviation in the number or constitution of the chromosomes (the tiny units containing the *genes* which determine and govern inherited physical and mental characteristics).

In psychiatry, aberration refers to emotional disturbances. *See also* ANOMALY; NEUROSIS.

**ABLATION,** surgical removal of a tumor, cancer, or other abnormal growth. *See* SURGERY.

**ABORTION,** in strictly medical language, means the interruption of a pregnancy and the loss of an unborn child during the first three months of pregnancy. It may be accidental, also called *spontaneous,* or it may be deliberate, or *induced.* After the third month, interruption of a pregnancy is called a *miscarriage.*

Induced abortion has long been one of the most controversial of all medical procedures. Many individuals object to the practice on religious or ethical grounds, and until recently, induced abortion was illegal throughout most of the United States except under certain circumstances. For example, in some states, induced abortion was permitted only if there was

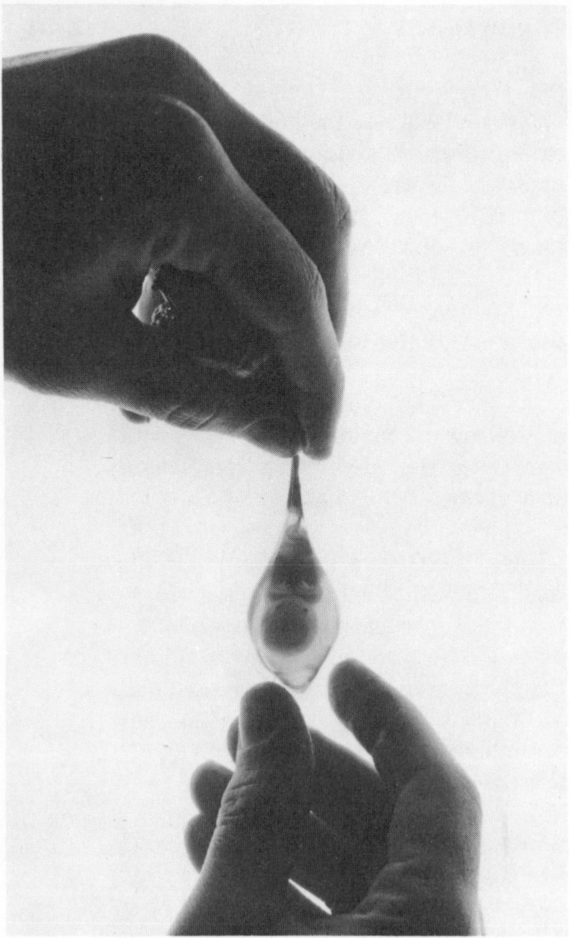

**Abortion**—This dramatic photograph shows an ectopic pregnancy—an embryo of 6–7 weeks in a Fallopian tube that was surgically removed from a woman. Weeks later, the growing fetus would have burst through the tube—resulting in death for the fetus and possibly fatal hemorrhaging in the mother. Performed for such an urgent medical reason, this is called a therapeutic abortion.

no other way to save the life of a woman. The main argument centers about whether an embryo or fetus is human, at what point it becomes human, the right to life of the unborn child, and the right of a woman to control her own body.

As increasing numbers of Americans supported legal, induced abortion, state laws began to be modified. By 1971, ten states allowed a woman to have an abortion "on demand." A year later, the U. S. Supreme Court decreed that abortion in the early months of pregnancy was a matter for the woman, not the law, to decide. The decision effectively weakened or overturned restrictive state laws.

Many abortions are induced for strictly medical reasons. These are called *therapeutic* abortions. One urgent medical reason is the presence of an ectopic pregnancy, a situation in which the embryo develops in the Fallopian tube instead of in the uterus. Such an embryo cannot survive. It will die and burst through the tube, endangering the mother's life, if it is not removed surgically. A woman who contracts German measles in early pregnancy may request an abortion because of the likelihood that her child will be malformed or mentally retarded. In cases of rape or incest, an induced abortion may be performed. A woman who has a severe heart, kidney, or blood ailment may require an abortion to save her health or life. A therapeutic abortion may be performed on a woman who already has several children and whose general health, age or both would make it difficult for her to have another and to care for her entire family properly. Lastly, special new procedures now make it possible to determine during pregnancy the presence of conditions such as Down's syndrome and Tay-Sachs disease. If one of these diseases, or another, should be detected, the woman may elect to have a therapeutic abortion rather than bear a child with serious physical or mental impairment.

The age of the fetus usually determines the technique used in induced abortion. During the first 12 weeks of pregnancy, dilatation and curettage (D and C) may be the preferred method. Dilatation refers to the stretching of the cervix in order to perform the curettage, or scraping of the walls. Alternatively, a suction apparatus may be used in early pregnancy to remove the embryo. When the pregnancy is more advanced, a strong salt solution is sometimes injected into the uterus to induce labor. It may be necessary to remove the entire uterus, or to cut into it through the abdomen to remove the larger fetus of a pregnancy in the fourth month or later.

If the pregnancy ends naturally before the fetus is sufficiently developed to live outside the body, the occurrence is called spontaneous abortion. As many as 15 percent of all pregnancies end this way between the fourth and twentieth weeks. In very early pregnancy, an imperfect fetus usually dies before it is aborted. A spontaneous abortion may be caused by excessive exertion or a bad fall. Other causes include infectious disease, glandular ailments, vitamin deficiency, and oxerexposure to x-rays. An abnormally developed uterus or inflammation of the lining of the uterus may end a pregnancy.

Bleeding, however slight, should always be reported to a physician, since it is the first sign of a spontaneous abortion. Pain in the back or abdomen may also be present. If a woman reports slight bleeding or other symptoms immediately, her doctor may be able to save her unborn infant.

If a spontaneous abortion does occur, the woman should be examined so that the doctor can determine whether all the contents of the uterus have been expelled. If the abortion is incomplete, he may have to perform a curettage of the uterus to remove the remaining placenta. *See also* ABORTION COMPLICATIONS; ABRUPTIO PLACENTAE; AMNIOCENTESIS; BLOOD TYPES; DILATATION AND CURETTAGE; GENETIC COUNSELING *and* **medigraphs** ECTOPIC PREGNANCY; GERMAN MEASLES; TAY-SACHS DISEASE; SYPHILIS.

▶ The Health of Women, *Conception and Contraception,* 1402. Sex and Sex Education, *Sex Education of Children,* 2643.

**ABORTION COMPLICATIONS,** often follow the interruption of a pregnancy by someone other than a physician. When induced abortions were almost always illegal and many women resorted to unlicensed persons, some of whom used crude techniques in unsanitary settings, abortion complications were frequent, and often fatal. Careless and ignorant methods can perforate the uterus and cause hemorrhage. Infection, kidney failure and shock are often associated with criminal abortion. If the uterus is punctured, abdominal surgery may be required to save the woman's life. Severe and protracted infection can cause the kidneys to stop functioning or to function imperfectly. In this situation, special dialysis equipment must be used to restore kidney function and prevent blood poisoning.

The chances of complications resulting from induced abortion are sharply reduced if the procedure is performed in a hospital or clinic by a physician.

**ABORTUS FEVER,** a communicable disease afflicting animals and humans. *See* UNDULANT FEVER.

**ABRASION,** a superficial injury to the skin or mucous membranes. A skinned knee or elbow are examples. Most abrasions come under the category of minor injuries, occurring in commonplace everyday situations. Nevertheless, abrasions should not be taken lightly, as they are highly susceptible to infection. Cleansing with soap and water is usually sufficient protection. If much bleeding or oozing of fluid takes place, the abraded area should be covered with sterile gauze after it is cleaned.

In dentistry, abrasion refers to the wearing away of tooth surface caused by chewing. *See also* FIRST AID.

**ABRUPTIO PLACENTAE,** premature separation of the placenta (afterbirth) before delivery of the fetus. The symptoms include vaginal bleeding, shock greater than that which might be due to the bleeding alone, and pain and tenderness in the abdomen. The mother may feel sudden violent movements of the fetus which indicate that it is being deprived of oxygen. The obstetrician should be called immediately to save the pregnancy. If the pregnancy cannot be saved, the uterus will have to be emptied of its contents. *See also* ABORTION; CHILDBIRTH; DILATATION AND CURETTAGE; PREGNANCY; PRENATAL CARE; VAGINA.

**ABSCESS,** a localized pocket of pus in a cavity formed by tissues that have broken down as the result of infection or injury. The inflamed area forming the cavity is red, painful, and swollen. An abscess is caused when bacteria enter a small wound, such as that caused by a splinter. White blood cells collect at the infected area to seal off the infection, to absorb the bacteria, and to liquefy them. The formation of thick yellowish pus results from this activity. The accumulating pus and the swelling of the inflamed tissues press against the nerves, creating pain. The redness is caused by a concentration of blood in the area. An abscess "comes to a head" as the wall of surrounding tissue becomes thin. When the abscess ruptures and the pus escapes, the pain and swelling subside.

A large, extremely painful abscess, such as a boil, should be professionally treated. A physician will open the abscess safely with a sterilized instrument and remove the pus without unnecessarily irritating the tissue. Even a small skin abscess should not be squeezed, since this is likely to spread the infection.

An abscess may form within the body as well as on the skin surface. They can occur, for example, in the chest, abdominal cavity, joints, glands, or at the root of a tooth. Sometimes, a doctor may have to cut into and drain an abscess to prevent its sac of infection from spreading into surrounding tissues or escaping into the bloodstream. If an abdominal abscess ruptures, the resulting general infection (called *peritonitis*) requires immediate emergency care. A widespread body infection, or *sepsis,* results from the emptying of an abscess into the bloodstream. *See also* BACTEREMIA; BLOOD; EMPYEMA; INFECTION; PYORRHEA *and* **medigraphs** APPENDICITIS AND PERITONITIS; CARBUNCLES, FURUNCLES AND FOLLICULITIS; LUNG ABSCESS; OSTEOMYELITIS; PILONIDAL CYST.

▶ The Importance of Skin, *Skin and Infection,* 2702.

◆ Battle Against Decay, 820.

**ABSORPTION,** the taking in of fluids or other substances by the skin, mucous membranes, or organs of the body. The absorbed material may be gaseous or fluid. Thus, the skin and mucous membranes—such as those lining the mouth and nose—absorb drugs applied on their surfaces. The digestive system absorbs solid and liquid foods. The large intestine absorbs fluid and the small intestine takes in carbohydrates, fats, and proteins for further absorption by the blood and distribution throughout the body.

◆ Burning Up the Food We Eat, 907.

**ABULIA,** loss or weakening of will power and the ability to make decisions. Abulia often occurs in certain mental illnesses, such as schizophrenia. *See also* SCHIZOPHRENIA.

**ACANTHOCYTOSIS,** a rare hereditary disorder characterized by skin and digestive disturbances, loss of muscular coordination, and mental retardation. These disturbances are believed to be due to faulty lipid (fat) utilization by the body. No specific treatment has been established. The disorder is also called *abetalipoproteinemia.*

**ACANTHOLYSIS,** a skin disturbance characterized by degeneration of the epidermal (outer skin) cells which occurs in the skin disease *pemphigus. See also* PEMPHIGUS.

**ACANTHOSIS,** a thickening of the inner layer of the skin, resulting in a horny growth on the surface. An acanthosis may vary in color from almost transparent to jet black. A doctor can burn off such a growth with a chemical or an electric cautery. *See also* KERATOSIS.

**ACAPNIA,** a condition in which the carbon dioxide content of the blood is below normal. *See also* BLOOD; CIRCULATORY SYSTEM.

**ACCESSORY SEX ORGANS,** organs which are related to the reproductive organs. In the male, the accessory sex organs include the *epididymis,* a portion of the seminal duct along the posterior border of the testis. Mature male sperm cells are stored here. The *prostate gland,* at the neck of the bladder, manufactures secretions that help transport the spermatozoa. In the female, the accessory sex organs include the *vulva,* two pairs of lip-shaped skin and soft membranes that surround the opening of the vagina, and the *clitoris,* a small projection of soft skin where the inner pair of vulva meet at the top. *See also* REPRODUCTIVE SYSTEM.

▶ Sex and Sex Education, *The Sexual Organs and Reproduction,* 2637.

**ACCIDENT PREVENTION.** More than half of all accidents occur on the highways and in the home. Preventive measures could significantly reduce the number of deaths and injuries.

*Preventing Highway Accidents.* Causes of highway deaths include speeding; fol-

**Accident Prevention**—No area should be overlooked when a home is made safe for a toddler. Crates and a small chair left in a back entry could lead to a bad fall for this little boy.

**Accident Prevention**—A baby should never be placed in bath water before being sure it is not too hot. Testing with the elbow gives a truer idea of water temperature than the hands.

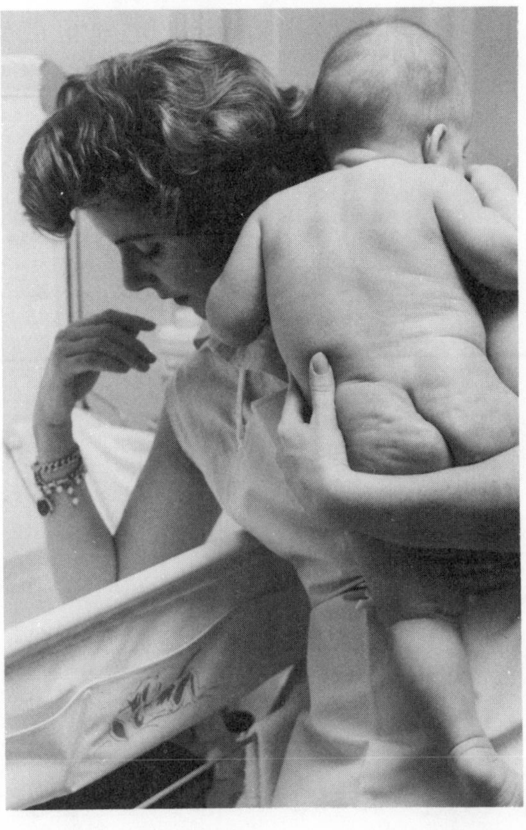

lowing too close; not paying attention to other vehicles, highway signs, and traffic signals; and failing to stay in the proper lane. Recklessness, emotional disturbance, impatience, and lack of consideration for other drivers are additional causes.

Almost two-thirds of all drivers involved in accidents have been drinking, and the use of drugs is being detected in an increasing number of accidents.

Following are several common sense suggestions for safer driving:

1. Know in advance what to do in an emergency.
2. Keep your car in good mechanical condition, with special attention to brakes, tires, lights, steering, shock absorbers, exhaust system, and windshield washers and wipers.
3. Do not exceed the legal speed limit. Judge road conditions and drive slower than the limit in bad weather or in poor lighting conditions.
4. Do not use alcohol or drugs before driving. Ask your doctor if any medications you are using could make you drowsy or slow down your reactions.
5. Do not drive if you are tired.

**Accident Prevention**—Good driving habits are the basis of a lifetime of safe driving. They can be instilled in new drivers only with serious lessons from an expert adult driver—preferably a professional instructor.

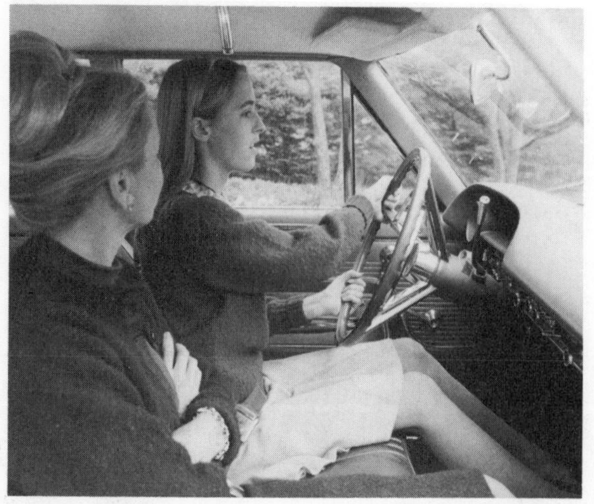

6. Drive defensively. Watch out for careless and speeding drivers, be careful at intersections even if you have the right of way, and be observant entering and leaving superhighway ramps.
7. Keep your emotions under control when you drive. An angry driver may swerve the steering wheel sharply or stamp down hard on the accelerator.
8. Do not allow passengers, pets, or packages to block your view. Do not permit horseplay in your car.
9. Keep your car ventilated at all times. This is especially important in cars that are closed much of the time, for heat in the winter and air-conditioning in the summer.
10. Have seat belts and put them on.

Within a ten-year period, the number of motorcycles in the United States increased 220 percent, about ten times the increase in the number of motor vehicles. Motorcyclists should take added precautions. The death rate for cyclists is about 30 per 100 million miles of motorcycle travel, compared with 5.7 deaths per 100 million miles of automobile travel. Cyclists should be specially trained, should wear protective clothing, including a helmet, and should regularly inspect their cycles.

*Preventing Home Accidents.* Most of the approximately 10,000 injuries each day in American homes are caused by carelessness or neglect. The most dangerous rooms are the kitchen and bathroom, but dark passageways, cellar stairs, and cluttered closets are also the scenes of accidents that result in injury or death.

THE FIRST SAFETY MEASURE homeowners should take to make their homes as accident-free as possible—and to teach their children safety habits—is to check the home carefully for safety hazards, and correct any that are found at once.

A careful tour of almost any home or apartment will turn up potentially dan-

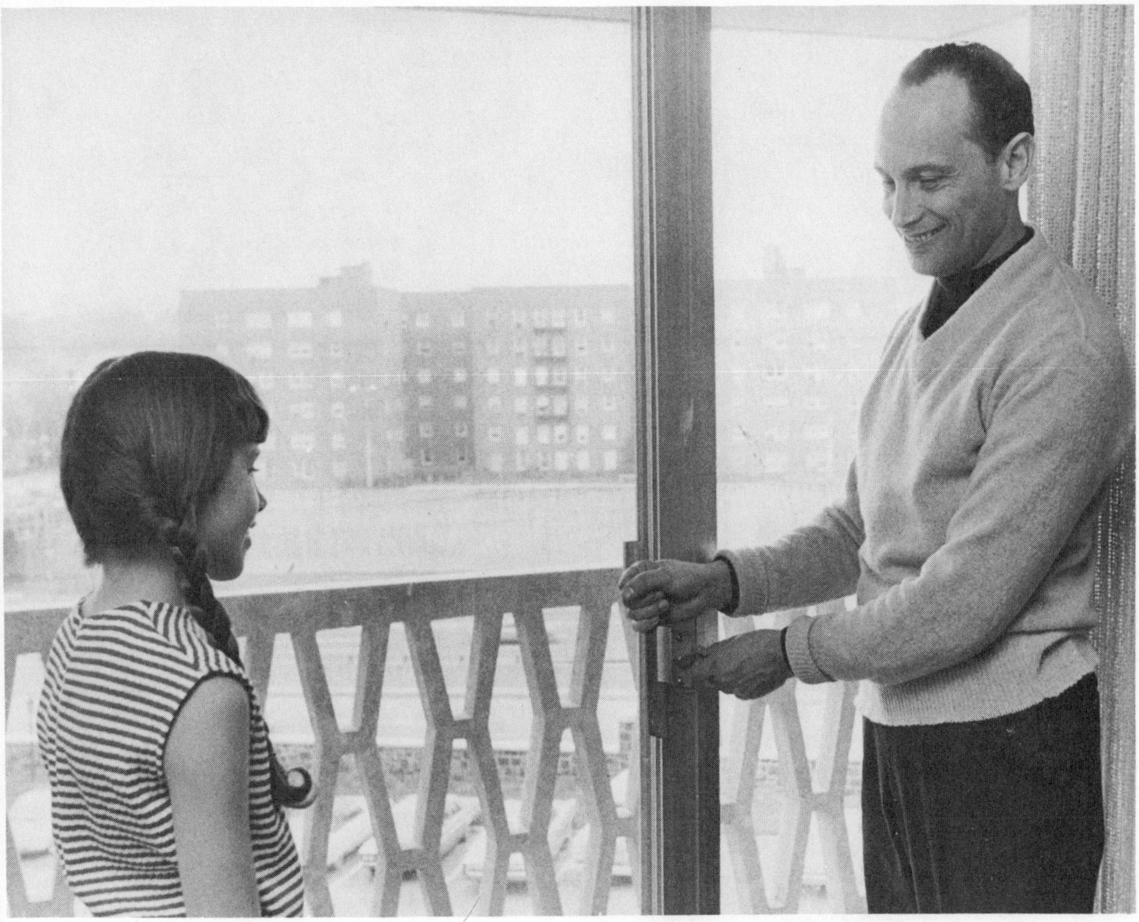

**Like so many people** in today's highly urbanized society, this father and daughter live in a high-rise apartment. A fall from the terrace could result in death or serious injury. The father wisely makes it a point to keep the door to the terrace locked when he is not around. He is also careful to instruct his oldest child in this procedure, so that younger children will be protected from mishaps about which they cannot yet be expected to understand. Right, this father wisely insists on the use of seat belts while driving. However careful a driver may be, an accident is always a possibility. The use of seat belts serves to minimize the extent of injuries sustained by preventing the occupant from impact with the windshield or dashboard in the event of collision with another motor vehicle or object. Many lives have been saved by the use of seat belts.

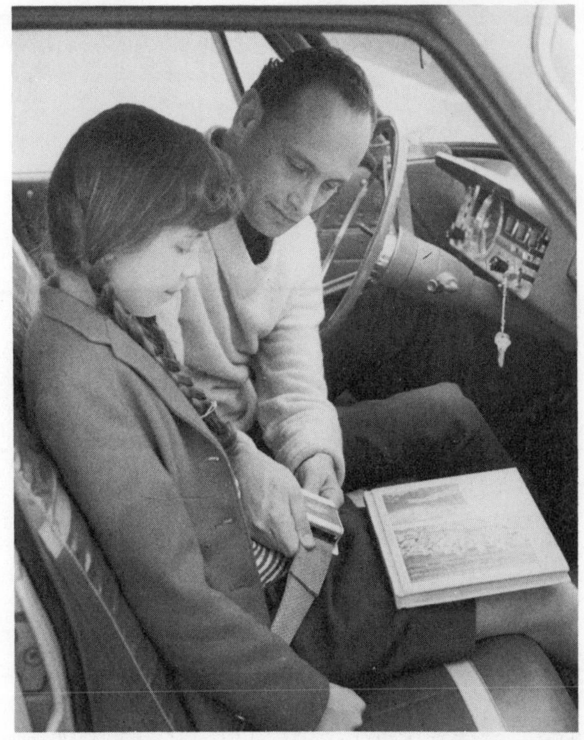

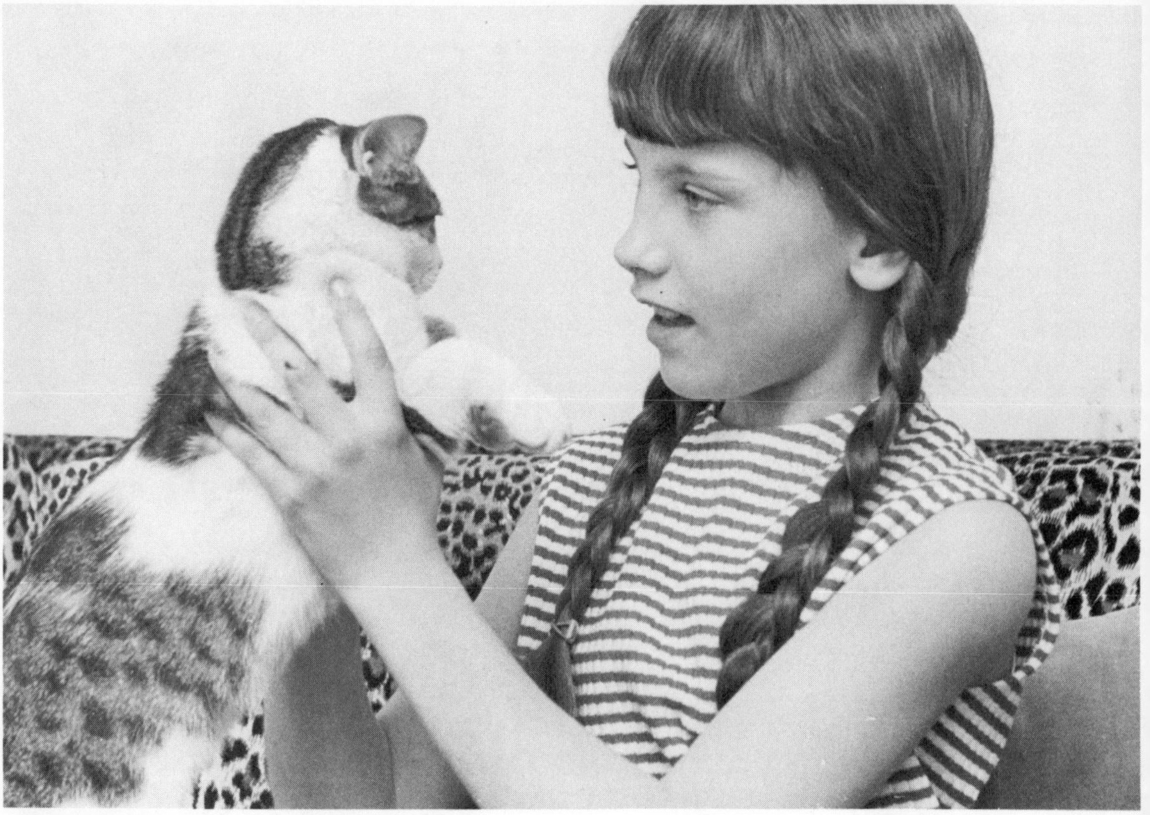

**Knowing how to deal** with pets is an important part of every child's safety education. The child above handles her cat gently. Treating a cat (or dog) roughly might provoke it to bite or scratch. In some cases, this could result in tetanus. This girl also has been taught that the proper way to carry scissors is with the blades pointing downwards *(below, left)*. In the family medicine chest *(below, right)*, potentially harmful drugs are kept on the top shelf.

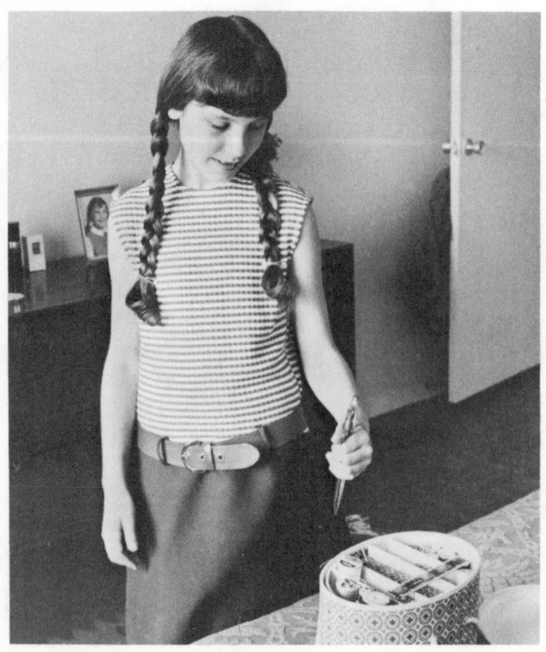

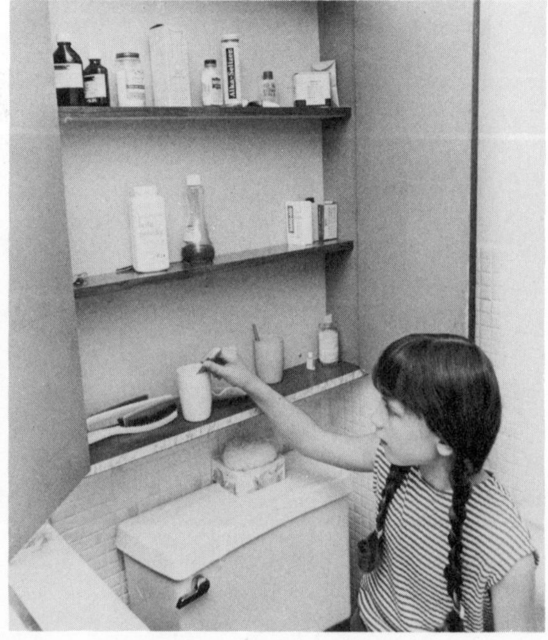

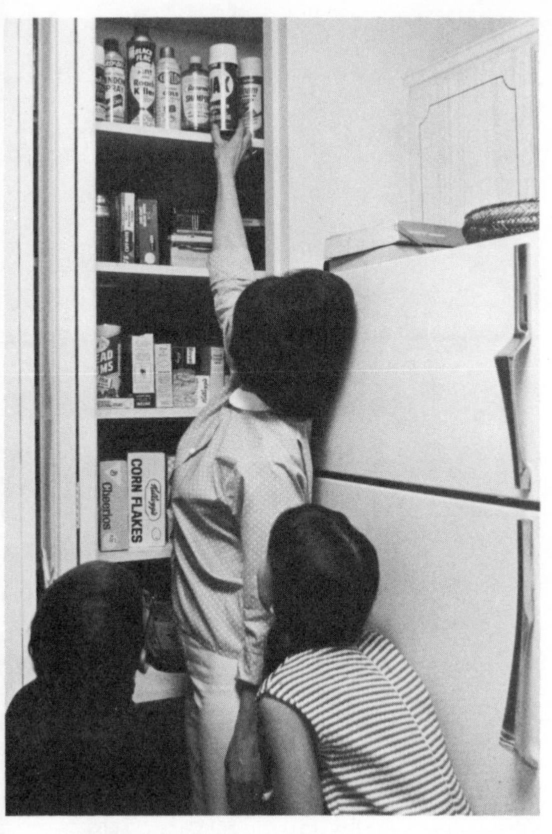


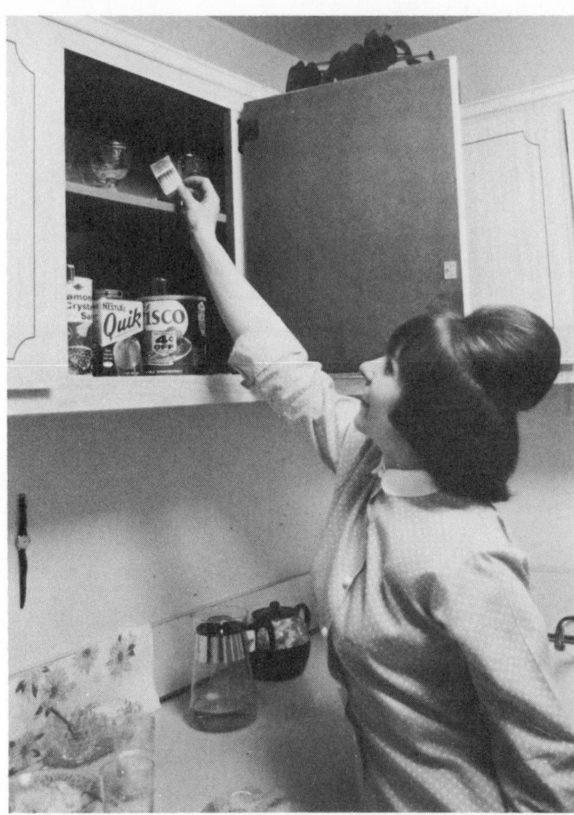


**Chemicals** which are clearly dangerous should always be kept well out of the reach of small children *(above, left)*. Poisoning accidents among children occur with distressing frequency and are easily preventable. Similarly, matches should be kept out of the reach of young children. Many of the household fires which take such a fearsome annual toll in lives and property are started by children too young and unaware to realize the consequences of their actions. Below, this mother takes the time to instruct her daughter in the proper procedure for peeling potatoes safely.

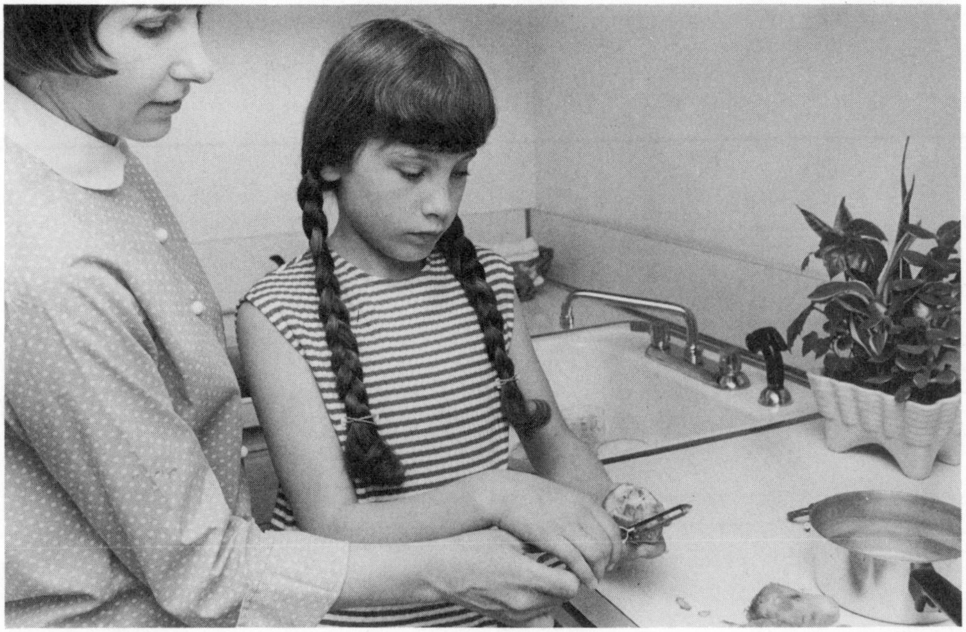

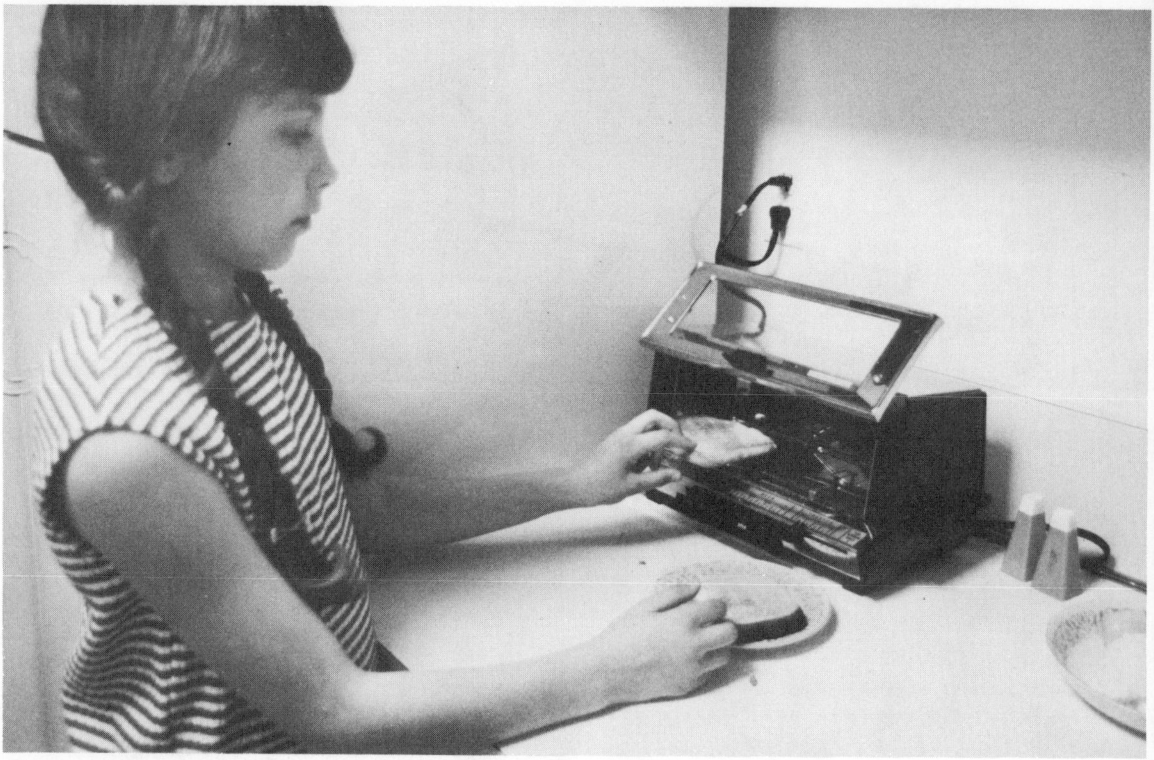

**Many of the commonest household** accidents occur in the kitchen. Careful observance of a few elementary safety rules can eliminate most of these mishaps. The use of a bread toaster in which all the operating mechanisms are visible may prevent many fingers from being burned. Safety rules should apply in the living room too. Television should be viewed from the proper distance in a room with contrasting light. Improper lighting may provoke problems of severe eyestrain.

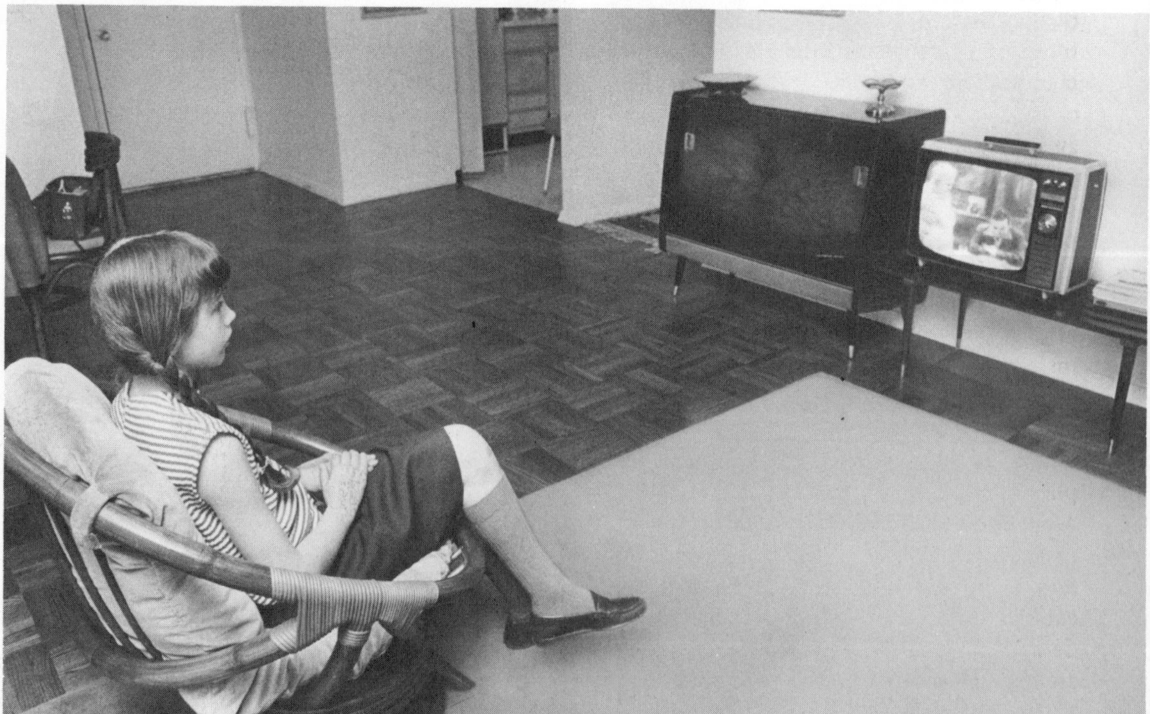

gerous situations. Outside, cracked and broken concrete should be replaced. Porches and steps should be kept in good condition. Entryways should be kept clear of children's toys and trash. Inside the home, stairs should have lights that can be controlled from both top and bottom, and hallways should be fitted with lighting receptacles at either end. The light switch for each room should be near the door, to avoid having to walk into a dark room to turn on a light. Small rugs on polished floors should be removed or fastened down securely with tacks, sprays, powders, or special mattings. Basement stairs should be kept in good repair and there should be a sturdy handrail. Basement storage should be neat; clutter is dangerous. Toys or other objects should never be left on any stairway in a house. Apartment hallways should be kept clear. If you have a basement locker in your apartment house, be sure it is kept locked and that it does not contain materials which could spontaneously ignite.

THE SECOND SAFETY MEASURE homeowners should take is to eliminate situations that are potentially hazardous to children in the home. Children—especially young children—are liable to cuts, swallowing dangerous drugs or poisons, falls, burns, electrical shock, and drowning. Following are some common sense preventive measures with which everyone should be familiar:

*Cuts.* Knives, scissors, and sharp tools attract children. Keep all sharp or pointed instruments out of your children's reach. They can learn about household devices and tools safely by handling, for example, blunt scissors and light wood or plastic tools.

*Medicines and Poisons.* Medicines tend to accumulate. Remove those that are no longer being used from the medicine cabinet, both because most medications deteriorate with age and because they create unnecessary clutter. All medicines should be carefully labeled and kept out of children's reach, preferably in a locked cabinet. Some medicines, like children's aspirin, are available in "child-resistant" packages that only an adult can open. But children are ingenious and strong. Common household items should also be safeguarded. Insecticides, cleaning agents, shoe polish, paint, paint thinner, kerosene, and other everyday substances can seriously harm or kill children. If a child is in a room that has its own gas or oil heater, a window must be kept open. As added preparation for emergencies, have the number of your local Poison Control Center posted at your telephone. Familiarize yourself with first aid remedies for the different types of poisons. If your child should swallow poison, do not induce vomiting if the poison is a caustic substance or a petroleum distillate such as kerosene. For other types of poison, *syrup of ipecac* and water should be administered at once to induce vomiting.

**Accident Prevention**—Children's play tools let them copy adult carpentry work without danger of hurting themselves. The serrated edges of this small hand saw have harmless blunt ends.

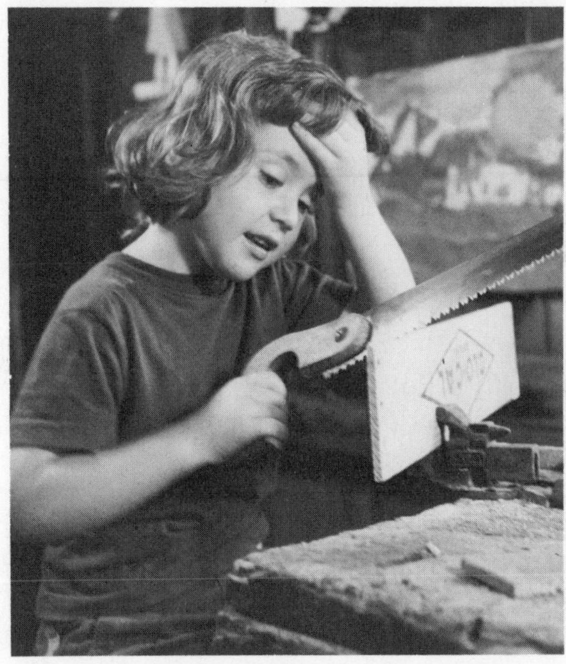

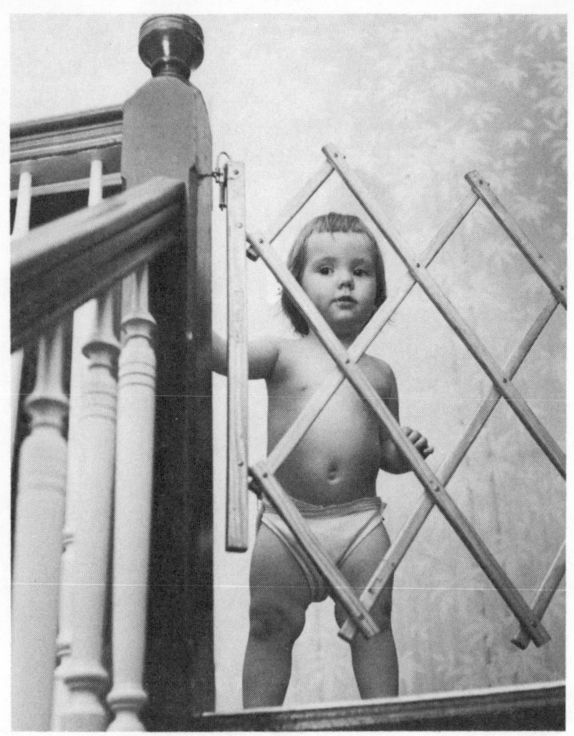

**Accident Prevention**—A tot's curiosity can lead to trouble. This type of gate at the top of a stairway protects the child from a bad tumble, but lets her watch the world below.

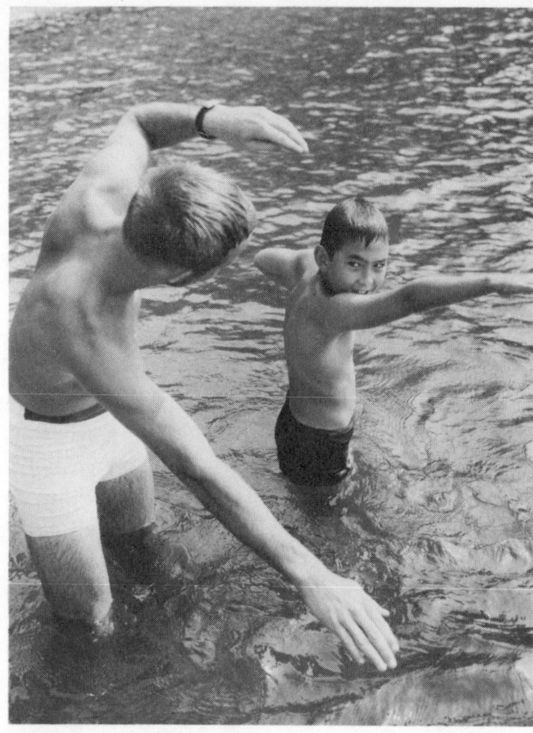

**Accident Prevention**—Swimming lessons, at as early an age as possible, are a must for safest enjoyment of this popular sport. Rescue and resuscitation courses are additional assets.

*Falls.* Floors should not be waxed heavily. Any spilled liquid should be removed immediately. A rubber mat in the bathtub or shower enclosure and a soft mat on the bathroom floor will cushion a fall. Rails on a baby's crib and playpen and on a child's bed should be secure. Windows on upper floors should have special locks to prevent them from being opened for more than a few inches. Stairs should be guarded at top and bottom by gates. New shoes should not be so slippery that running and climbing become unsafe. Carpets on waxed floors should be installed so that they cannot slip. Elderly people should stay off ladders.

*Burns.* Turn handles of pots and pans so that they do not project into the room and into a child's line of vision. Fireplaces should be completely screened when they are in use. Matches and cigarette lighters should not be left where children can reach them. A young child should not be left alone in a bathtub even for an instant, both because he may turn on the hot water faucet and because of the danger of drowning.

*Electrical shock.* Close unused wall sockets with blank plugs. Use special flat plugs for lamps and electrical appliances; they are much less easily pried out of the socket. Children must learn never to touch a wall switch or electric appliance when their hands or any other parts of their bodies are wet. These and other safety measures can be taught in a positive way, so that children learn how to handle electrical devices safely. They should not be made afraid of their environment.

*Drowning.* Hardly anyone would leave an infant in its bath unattended, but some parents take a chance, "just for a second," with children two or three years old. Young children should not be left alone in their bath. Nor should they be allowed to play in a sinkful of water if any electrical appliance is within reach. Safe water play should be encouraged, however, always with a parent or older child available, so that young children will not be frightened when they are first taken to the swimming pool, backyard splash pool, lake, or ocean.

THE THIRD MAJOR SAFETY MEASURE is to teach children about hazardous situations outside the home. Learning about traffic is most important. Boys and girls must learn how and when to cross streets, and why they should watch for oncoming vehicles even if they are crossing with the green light. City children should play in parks and playgrounds. Parents should warn their children against playing in the streets, especially in heavily trafficked streets. When high school students learn to drive, they will already have acquired safe driving standards if their parents have set good safety examples.

Older children and adolescents enjoy using hand tools, power equipment, and garden appliances such as power mowers. They should be taught to use them safely. Power saws, drills, lathes, and other basement equipment can seriously hurt an individual. A power mower should never be used by a barefoot operator. The area to be mowed should be kept clean of sharp objects and rocks that a mower can pick up and project with the speed of a bullet, directly at the user. Do-it-yourself enthusiasts should carefully inspect the ladders they plan to use. Never permit anyone to substitute a box or chair for a ladder.

*Firearms.* Millions of Americans now have firearms in their homes, and more than half the 2800 accidental deaths due to firearms yearly occur in the home, not in the field. Children should never be allowed to touch any firearm. Parents who want their adolescent children to know how to handle them should always act as though the firearms were loaded. Anyone using a handgun or rifle should know thoroughly how it works, its safety fea-

**Accident Prevention**—Boy Scouts precisely and carefully lay the groundwork for a campfire. They know that resourcefulness goes hand in hand with application of the rules for safety.

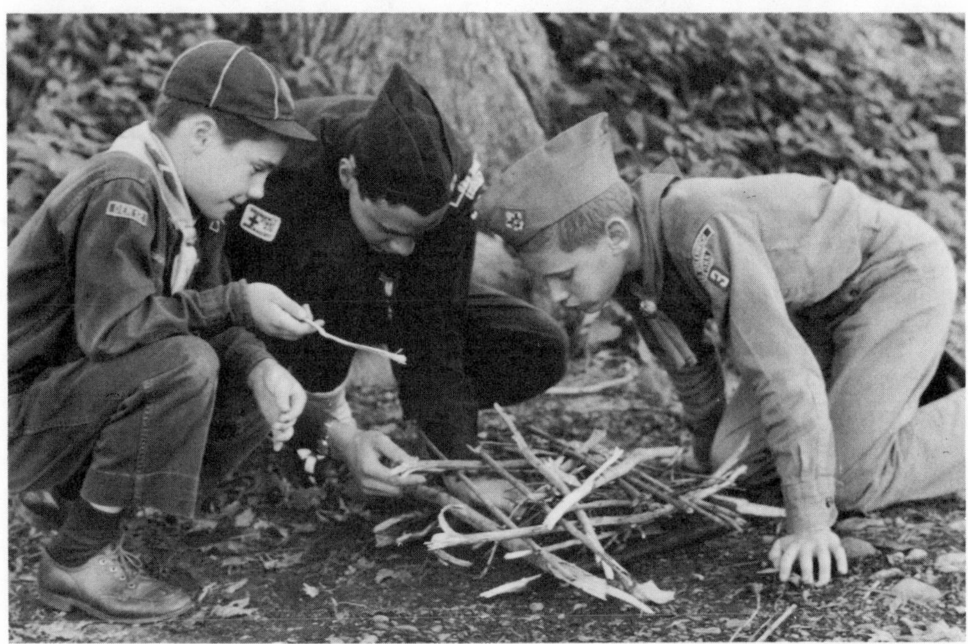

tures, and its hazards. Under no circumstances should anyone, adult or teenager, treat a firearm as though it were a toy.

In summary, preventing accidents is a job for adults. They must protect infants and young children, teach their children accident prevention methods, and teach them common sense, confidence, and responsibility. *See also* ACCIDENT-PRONE; DROWNING; FIRST AID; RESUSCITATION.

▶ Vision Impairment, *How to Keep Your Sight,* 2952.

◆ Scaling the Heights, 189. Road Accident, 1243.

**ACCIDENT-PRONE,** term used to describe people who have many more accidents than is average for people of comparable age and occupation. Often, their accidents recur at the same time of the month, week, or even hour. The accidents are more frequent in summer than at other times of the year and are often associated with emotional stress. Frequently, people who seem to be accident-prone have fewer accidents after attaining maturity; but some appear to remain accident-prone throughout life. *See also* ACCIDENT PREVENTION.

**ACCOMMODATION,** the ability of the lens of the eye to adjust itself for viewing near or distant objects. For distance vision, the pupils of the eye become large, the lens flattens, and they direct away from each other. The process is reversed for close vision. After about the age of 40, the lenses begin to harden and the ability of the eye to accommodate diminishes. Special glasses may be required for close vision. Glasses may be fitted with bifocals (two lenses in one) or trifocals (three lenses in one) to help a middle-aged or older person accommodate his vision. *See also* EYE; FARSIGHTEDNESS; NEARSIGHTEDNESS.

**ACETEST,** the commercial name for a small kit that can be used in the home by diabetics to test for *acetone* in the urine. The presence of acetone is a symptom of *acidosis,* a condition that should be called to the attention of a physician immediately. *See also* ACETONE; ACIDOSIS *and* **medigraph** DIABETES.

**ACETIC ACID,** a colorless liquid that gives vinegar its sour taste. *Glacial acetic acid,* which contains 99.5 per cent acetic acid, and *trichloroacetic acid,* a more dilute form, are used as caustics to remove warts. The more dilute concentrations of acetic acid are used to rid the hair of nits, in *pediculosis* (head lice).

**ACETONE,** a colorless liquid normally found in small quantities in the blood and urine. An increase in acetone is dangerous for diabetics. A test for excessive acetone is as important as the test for sugar in the blood. *See also* ACETEST *and* **medigraph** DIABETES.

**ACETYLSALICYLIC ACID,** the scientific term for *aspirin.* Aspirin has been used since 1893 to relieve pain and reduce fever. Aspirin does not cure any illness, but it may prevent the serious brain damage that an exceptionally high fever can cause. Aspirin does not interfere with the body's ability to fight a disease. Large amounts of aspirin are fatal to infants, and adult doses can induce intestinal bleeding in children. Exactly how aspirin works in the body is still unknown. For persons who suffer digestive symptoms when taking aspirin, equally effective substitutes are available. *See also* ANALGESIA; MEDICINE CHEST.

**ACHALASIA,** the failure of the smooth muscle fibers of the gastrointestinal tract to relax where they join with another part of the tract. Achalasia can cause an enlargement of the portion of the digestive tract above the affected area. *See also* COLON; DIGESTION; DIGESTIVE SYSTEM.

**ACHARD-THIERS SYNDROME,** a disorder in diabetic women characterized by development of excessive hair on the face and chin. The condition is also called *virilism.* Women with this syndrome often have changes of the voice and menstrual difficulties. Their breasts get smaller, they gain weight, and the clitoris enlarges.

Achard-Thiers syndrome may be associated with enlargement of the adrenal glands and with excess androgenic (male) hormones in the bloodstream. In drastic cases, surgical removal of the adrenal glands may be required; the woman must then, however, take for life the hormones normally manufactured by the *adrenal cortex,* as these are essential to life. *See also* ADRENAL GLAND; ADRENAL GLAND DISORDERS; VIRILISM.

**ACHE,** a dull, constant, sometimes throbbing pain. A backache often is described as a dull pain, and a toothache or headache as a throbbing pain. A dull aching pain of the bones occurs in influenza, and muscular rheumatism involves aching of the muscles.

An ache, like all other types of pain, is useful and even life-saving. It is a warning signal, indicating that something is wrong. Without the ache of a strained back, a decayed tooth, a bruised muscle, or an inflamed joint, a person would not know that something was wrong until much more damage had been done.

How quickly a person feels pain and how much he or she can tolerate is both physiological and psychological. The *pain threshold* is a measure of the stimulus needed in order to register pain. The ability to sustain pain without complaining, crying, or inability to work varies greatly from person to person.

Aching—possibly caused by the build-up of toxic substances—often follows strenuous exercise. The achiness gradually disappears with rest. The same aching feeling accompanies many illnesses, including a severe cold and malfunctioning kidneys. In such illnesses, the accumulation of wastes in the system produce the symptom of generalized aching until the illness disappears or is successfully treated. *See also* ACETYLSALICYLIC ACID; ANALGESIA; NERVOUS SYSTEM; PAIN *and* **medigraphs** MIGRAINE HEADACHE; RHEUMATOID ARTHRITIS.

**ACHILLES TENDON,** the strong prominent tendon at the back of the heel, connecting the calf muscles to the heel bone. Tapping the Achilles tendon normally

**Achilles Tendon**—This band of tough fibrous tissue attaches the calf muscle to the heel bone. When the muscle is flexed, the tendon lifts the heel and accomplishes a vital movement of walking. It is one of the most prominent and best known tendons of the body.

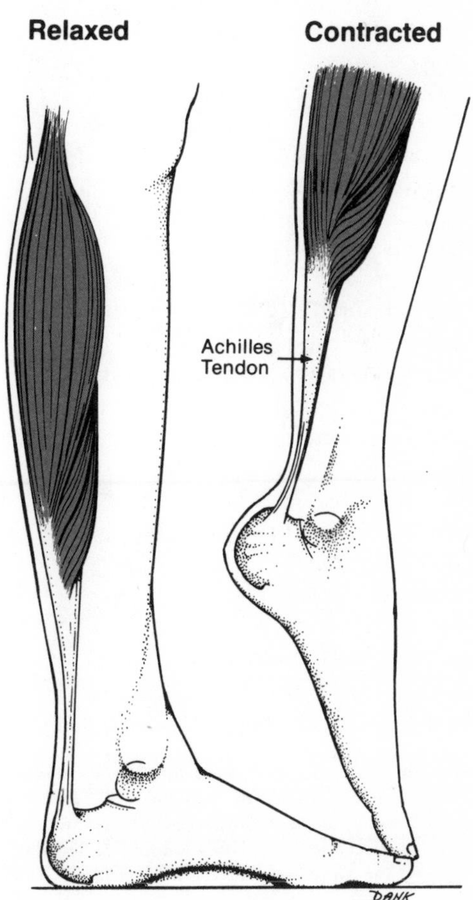

produces an ankle jerk, or reflex. If this reflex is missing or if it is exaggerated, disease or injury of the nerves of the leg muscles or the spinal cord may exist. The name derives from Homer's *Iliad,* in which Achilles was vulnerable only in his heel, the one part of his body which remained dry when his mother dipped him in the River Styx in the belief that this would render him impervious to injury. *See also* MUSCLE.

**ACHLORHYDRIA,** the absence of *hydrochloric acid* in the gastrointestinal juices. Hydrochloric acid aids digestion by activating the enzyme *pepsin* in the stomach, and by breaking down foods into components that can be absorbed by the blood. Complete achlorhydria is rare, occurring only in about ten percent of patients with stomach disorders. Persons with a less than normal secretion of hydrochloric acid may have few digestive symptoms, or none at all. However, achlorhydria is sometimes a symptom of serious disease, such as cancer or destruction of the stomach lining by inflammation. *Pernicious anemia* is associated with achlorhydria. *See also* ABDOMINAL PAIN; ANEMIA; DIGESTION; HYDROCHLORIC ACID *and* **medigraph** PERNICIOUS ANEMIA.

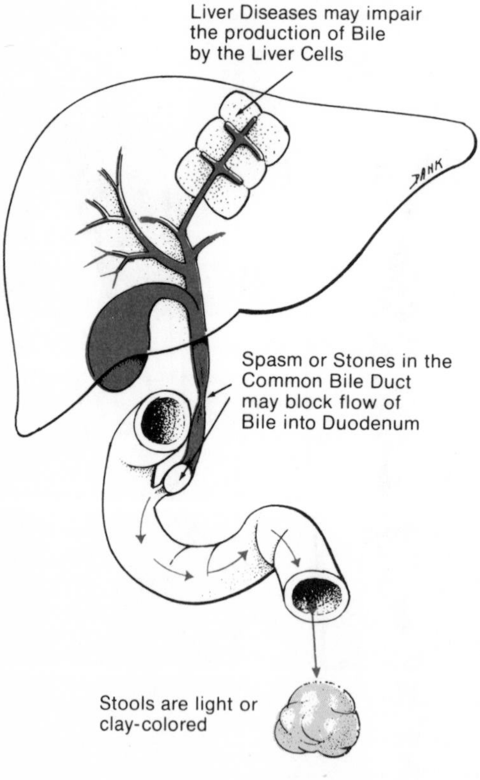

Liver Diseases may impair the production of Bile by the Liver Cells

Spasm or Stones in the Common Bile Duct may block flow of Bile into Duodenum

Stools are light or clay-colored

**Acholia**—Lack of bile flowing into the duodenum causes serious digestive problems. It can be caused by insufficient production of bile by the liver or blockage in the duct leading to the duodenum. The condition can require surgery.

**ACHOLIA,** a condition that occurs when *bile* cannot flow normally into the small intestine, due to an obstruction of the bile duct from the liver. This situation seriously impairs digestion and may be critical. Surgery is often required to relieve the obstruction. *See also* BILE; LIVER.

**ACHONDROPLASIA,** a disturbance of the growth process that produces a type of *dwarfism.* The condition is congenital, beginning with the growth of the embryo. The torso is usually normal, but the head is disproportionately large and the arms and legs are smaller than normal and curved. Most infants with this ailment are stillborn. In those who survive, mental and sexual development and life expectancy are not affected. Their muscles generally are stronger than those of normal individuals. A dwarf is different from a *midget,* whose body proportions are normal although the entire body is unusually small. Achondroplasia is an abnormal development of the embryo that affects the growth of the bones. Other growth disturbances are caused by nutritional or hormonal deficiencies. *See also* DWARFS; GENETIC COUNSELING.

**ACHROMYCIN,** a trademark for *tetracycline,* an antibiotic. Achromycin is effective against many types of bacteria and is among the safest of antibiotics. *See also* ANTIBIOTICS.

**ACHYLIA,** a complete lack of gastric juices from the stomach. The same term is sometimes used to describe a lack of secretions from the pancreas. An extremely rare condition, it may be associated with a wasting away of the lining of the stomach. *See also* DIGESTION; HYDROCHLORIC ACID; PANCREAS; STOMACH *and* **medigraph** PANCREATITIS.

**ACID,** a large and diverse group of chemicals, both organic and inorganic, having the common properties of a sour taste, solubility in water, and the release of hydrogen ions in solution. Mineral, or inorganic acids, include hydrochloric, nitric, and sulfuric. The organic group includes citric, lactic, and uric acids. A simple test for an acid is to put a small quantity on litmus paper, which acid turns from blue to red.

Many acids play important roles in the chemical processes that are a normal and vital part of the functions of body cells and tissues. *Amino acids* are the fundamental units of proteins. *Ascorbic acid* (*vitamin C*), found in citrus fruits, tomatoes, and many vegetables, is an essential part of a balanced diet. A disturbance of the acid content of the body can lead to serious disease. For example, a high level of *uric acid* produces gout.

Some inorganic acids corrode human tissues. Taken internally, they seriously damage the mouth, throat, esophagus, and stomach. If they enter the larynx, they will interfere with breathing. Antidotes for acid poisoning include large doses of milk of magnesia, milk, soapy water, or egg whites. Hot-water sponges and moist compresses applied to the throat will aid breathing and hot moist applications on the abdominal area can relieve stomach pains. If the skin is burned by sulfuric or nitric acid, the burned area should be washed immediately with diluted baking soda solution (4 tablespoons of baking soda in a quart of water), then bathed continuously with the soda solution. Basically, first-aid treatment for acid burns involves the neutralization of the affected area by an alkali, the chemical reverse of an acid. If an acid is swallowed, vomiting should *not* be induced, since this will burn the esophagus and throat a second time. *See also* BURNS; CITRIC ACID; ELECTROLYTES; HYDROCHLORIC ACID; NIACIN; URIC ACID; VITAMINS *and* **medigraphs** GOUT; PELLAGRA; SCURVY.

◆ Acids and Alkalis, 1608.

**ACIDOSIS,** the tendency toward overacidity that characterizes certain diseases. The blood is normally slightly alkaline, and is so maintained by blood chemicals and by the action of the lungs and kidneys in removing waste products. Uncorrected acidosis causes disorientation, coma, and death.

When extensive loss of fluid results from vomiting or diarrhea, so much alkaline substance may be lost that acidosis develops. The most readily recognized symptoms of acidosis are headache, weakness, rapid breathing, and a fruity odor on the breath. Laboratory tests enable a doctor to make a precise diagnosis of the acid-alkaline balance. The treatment for acidosis consists of replacing the lost fluid—by mouth if possible and by injection into the tissues or veins if necessary—and then determining the basic cause of the condition and implementing appropriate remedial measures.

*Diabetes* is the most common disorder in which acidosis occurs. The body of a diabetic cannot metabolize sugar, so that fats are incompletely burned and acid substances are produced. The body must then develop alkaline substances to neutralize them. *Poisons, diseases,* or *injuries* can produce acidosis—for example, aspirin, antifreeze, and rubbing alcohol poisoning; kidney failure; and diarrhea.

Certain foods are associated with acid formation, including lean beef, white bread, chicken, egg yolk, oysters, veal, wheat, pork, and fish. Alkaline-producing foods include tomatoes, prunes, carrots, lima beans, oranges, lemons, cantaloupe, lettuce, peaches, potatoes, and dried peas. Anyone maintaining a balanced diet need not worry that eating any of these foods will disturb the acid-alkaline balance of his body. Digestive distress, including belching and heartburn, is often blamed on "acid," but the problem may lie in the gallbladder or in the intestinal tract. A stomach ulcer may be responsible. Certain heart conditions may also cause symptoms that the sufferer describes as "indigestion." Consistent "acid stomach" is a signal to consult a doctor. *See also* COMA; INSULIN *and* **medigraph** DIABETES.

# ACNE

ACNE IS A CONDITION IN WHICH inflammation and infection of the *sebaceous* (oil) *glands* and *ducts* results in pimples, pustules and cysts on the skin.

### causes

The underlying cause of acne, which to one degree or another affects approximately 80 percent of all teenagers, is the glandular revolution that takes place with the onset of puberty. At this time, the pituitary governor of glandular activity alters the proportion of the male sex hormone *androgen* and the female sex hormone *estrogen* so that sexual *maturation* can be accomplished. Between puberty and maturity, both boys and girls have a consistently high level of androgen. This temporary increase in the androgen level stimulates the production of the sebaceous glands which ordinarily discharge the fluid secretion *sebum* through the pores for lubricating the skin. Overproduction of sebum causes it to turn into a paste which backs up and plugs up the ducts extending from the glands in the underlying derma through the layers of the epidermis.

### symptoms

Since the skin pores are tiny and often clogged by dirt or cosmetics, the fatty sebum accumulates under the skin and forms a pimple, a whitehead or a blackhead. These manifestations of acne are most likely to appear on the parts of the body where the glands are most numerous—particularly around the nose, the cheeks and the shoulders. The dark color of the characteristic blackheads is not the result of dirt, but of the discoloring effect of air on the fatty substance in the clogged pore. Bacteria on the skin surface may eat their way through the pasty accumulation into the ducts and the derma itself causing not only pimples in which pus gathers but, in severe cases, cysts that damage underlying tissue.

### treatment

In a majority of cases, acne is a transitory condition that gradually diminishes with the stabilization of hormones in adulthood. In its mild form, it can usually be controlled by a rigorous routine of cleanliness and the avoidance of rich desserts, fried foods and cola beverages. Creams and cosmetics that further clog the pores should be eliminated in favor of medicated soap and hot water. Sun lamp treatments and medications containing vitamin A may be used under a doctor's supervision. Pimples should not be "squeezed" since this method of eliminating pus can lead to more serious infection.

Severe cases of acne that leave the skin pitted and scarred require professional

# Acne

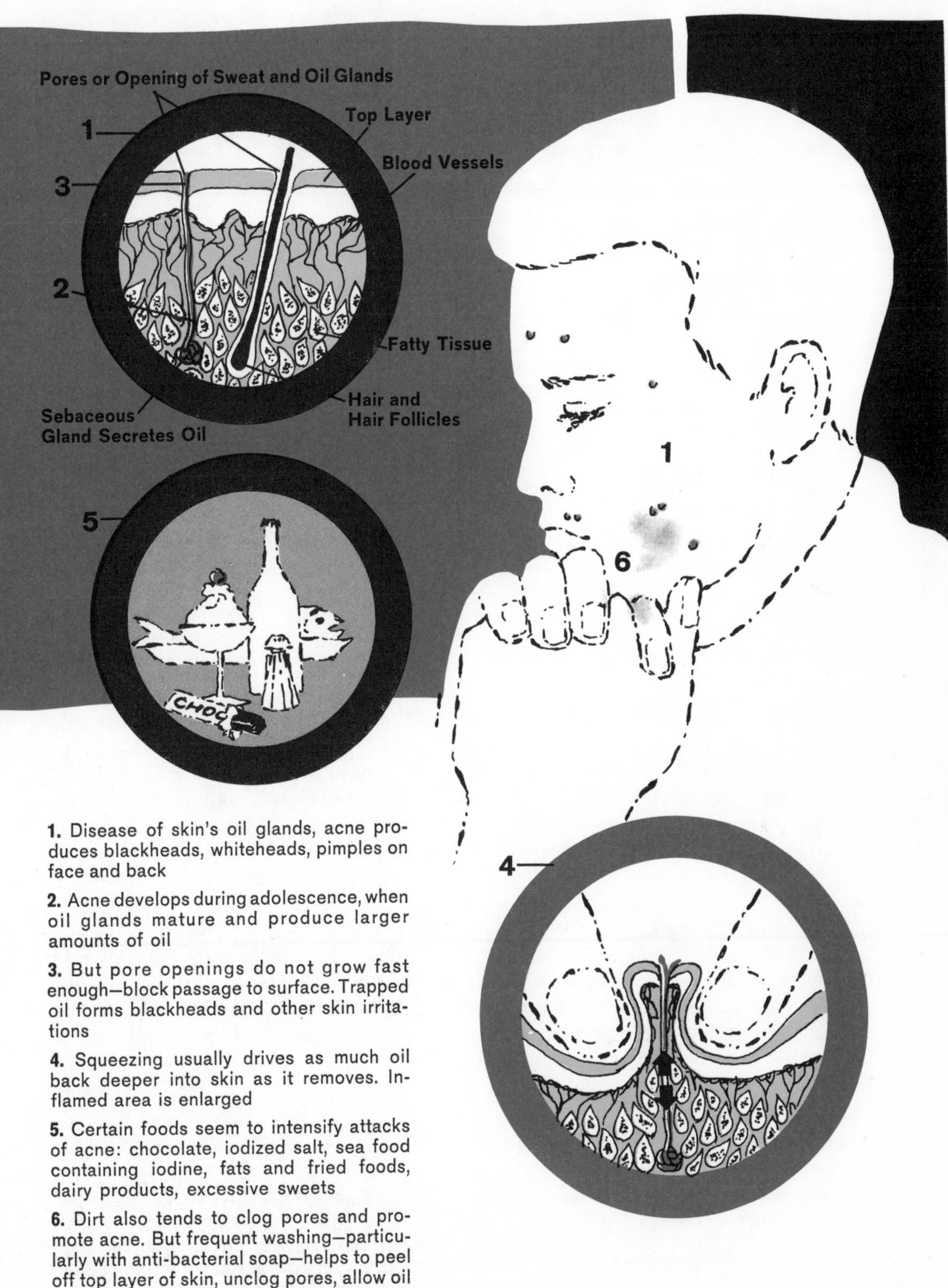


**1.** Disease of skin's oil glands, acne produces blackheads, whiteheads, pimples on face and back

**2.** Acne develops during adolescence, when oil glands mature and produce larger amounts of oil

**3.** But pore openings do not grow fast enough—block passage to surface. Trapped oil forms blackheads and other skin irritations

**4.** Squeezing usually drives as much oil back deeper into skin as it removes. Inflamed area is enlarged

**5.** Certain foods seem to intensify attacks of acne: chocolate, iodized salt, sea food containing iodine, fats and fried foods, dairy products, excessive sweets

**6.** Dirt also tends to clog pores and promote acne. But frequent washing—particularly with anti-bacterial soap—helps to peel off top layer of skin, unclog pores, allow oil to emerge, and fights bacterial inflammation

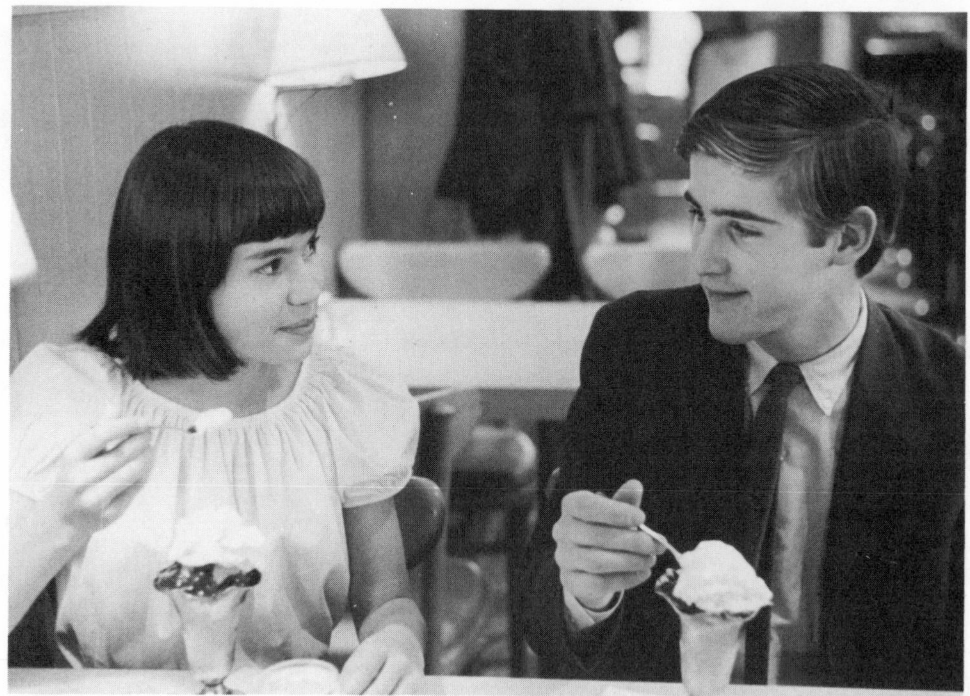

**Acne**—Sundaes and other rich desserts are best avoided by teenagers who have acne. The skin condition results from increased production of the skin's oil glands that occurs with hormonal changes at puberty. Fats and fried foods may also cause flareups of this embarrassing skin problem.

attention. The technique of *dermabrasion,* in which high-speed rotary wire brushes remove the outer layer of damaged skin, produces satisfactory results in many instances. It should not be undertaken unless a qualified dermatological specialist has been consulted.

Adolescents are especially sensitive about their appearance and should not be teased about their pimples. A youngster whose emotional well-being is seriously threatened by skin problems may require a few sessions with a sympathetic psychotherapist for the necessary reassurance that acne in most cases is only a temporary condition.

▶ The Importance of Skin, *Skin and Appearance,* 2689, *Skin and Inheritance,* 2696; *Skin and Foods,* 2698; *Skin and Adolescence,* 2708.

**ACNE ROSACEA.** *See* ROSACEA.

**ACONITE,** a brownish-orange drug derived from the root of *monkshood,* once used medically to slow the heart action, reduce temperature, and ameliorate pain. If taken inadvertently, it acts as a poison, causing a tingling sensation in the mouth, a burning pain in the stomach, weakened pulse, slower breathing rate, and a cold wet skin. First-aid treatment for aconite poisoning is to make the person vomit by giving him a tablespoon of mustard in a glass, of water. He should be put in bed, kept warm, and massaged. He should be encouraged to drink plenty of hot coffee. A doctor should be called immediately.

**ACOUSTIC NERVE,** the eighth *cranial nerve,* related to hearing and to the sense of balance. Symptoms of some neurological ailments are associated with this nerve, among them loss of hearing, ringing in the ears, dizziness, and disequilibrium. *See also* AUDITORY NERVE; EAR; HEARING; NERVOUS SYSTEM; RINGING IN THE EARS; VERTIGO *and* **medigraph** MÉNIÈRE'S DISEASE.

**ACQUIRED HEMOLYTIC ANEMIA.** When there is increased destruction of the red blood cells, it is called hemolytic anemia. When this condition is not inherited, but is caused by some other factor, it is called *acquired* hemolytic anemia. The causes include poisons, hypersensitivity to certain drugs, and other diseases. *See also* ANEMIA.

**ACRIFLAVINE,** once used as an antiseptic and in the treatment of gonorrhea. It has been superseded by a broad range of antibiotics. Acriflavine is an orange-yellowish crystalline substance, derived from coal tar.

**ACROCYANOSIS,** a disorder of the hands—and, less commonly, the feet—characterized by a bluish discoloration (*cyanosis*), profuse sweating, and occasionally swelling. The condition is often associated with *emotional stress* and *asthenic personality*. Sometimes, disorders of the *endocrine glands* may be involved.

Protection from cold is usually sufficient treatment (unless there are underlying endocrine abnormalities, in which case they must be specifically treated). Occasionally, *tolazoline* or *nicotinyl alcohol* may be given orally to dilate the blood vessels.

**ACRODYNIA,** a disease of infants and young children, up to about three years of age. Its characteristics are swollen, bluish-red hands and feet, muscular pains, and disordered digestion. A child suffering with acrodynia becomes generally sluggish, physically and mentally. Contact with *mercury* can cause acrodynia. Mercury and its compounds are found in some paints and in certain ointments. Children eating paint chips may suffer this form of mercury poisoning, as well as the better-known lead poisoning. Acrodynia is not contagious but it may last for months. It can be treated successfully. However, if treatment is delayed, permanent brain damage may occur. Generalized arthritis is also a possible complication. This ailment is also called *pink disease* because of its characteristic red skin rash. *See also* **medigraph** MERCURY POISONING.

## ACROMEGALY AND GIANTISM

ACROMEGALY AND GIANTISM are disturbances of the growth process affecting bone and muscle development to the point where an adult victim can attain a height of eight to nine feet and a weight of 500 pounds.

### causes

The two conditions are the result of oversecretion of the growth-stimulating hormone *somatotrophin* by the anterior lobe of the *pituitary gland*. When the glandular disorder occurs in adulthood, it is often caused by a slowly developing tumor in the area.

### symptoms

When the pituitary oversecretion begins in childhood, the resulting condition is called *giantism* or *gigantism*. It is characterized by overgrowth of the long bones of the skeleton, and overdevelopment of the musculature and internal organs. Abnormal height and grotesquely large hands and feet are manifest before adulthood.

## **Acromegaly and Giantism** (Diseases of Overactive Pituitary Gland)

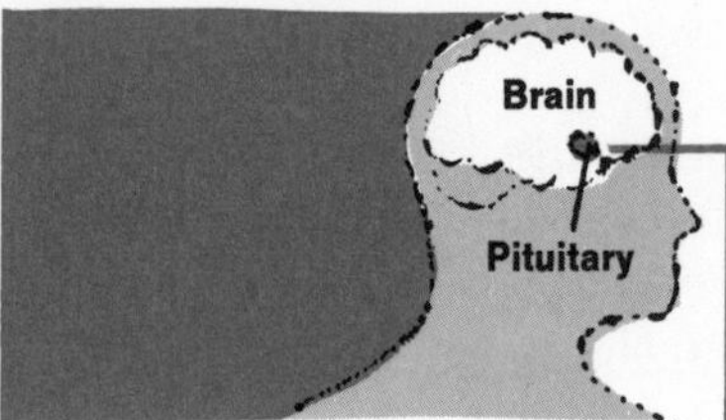


Tumor of anterior pituitary gland results in overproduction of hormones controlling growth

If tumor becomes active . . .

after normal growth years . . .

**Acromegaly**

With growth no longer possible in long bones, excessive growth slowly takes place in other areas:

**1.** Soft tissues—lips, tongue, ears, nose

**2.** Bony structure—protruding lower jaw, spade-like hands, enlarged feet, hunched back

**3.** Disturbance of sexual functions—impotence in men, ceasing of menstruation in women

**4.** Other possible complications—diabetes, visual disturbances and blindness, loss of strength

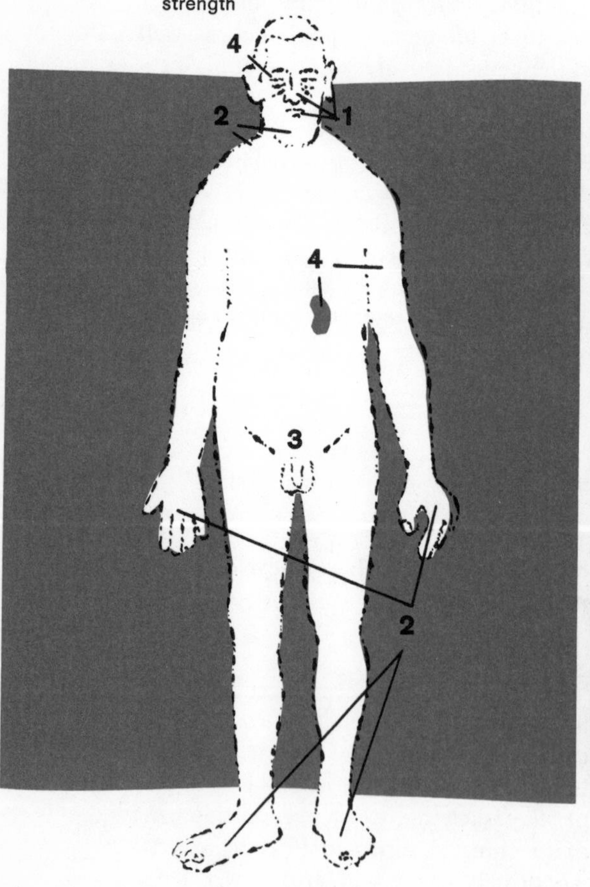


before normal growth years . . .

**Giantism**

**1.** Long bone growth continues, resulting in well proportioned giant 7-8 feet tall

**2.** However, if not arrested, gigantism may progress to stage of increasing weakness and death

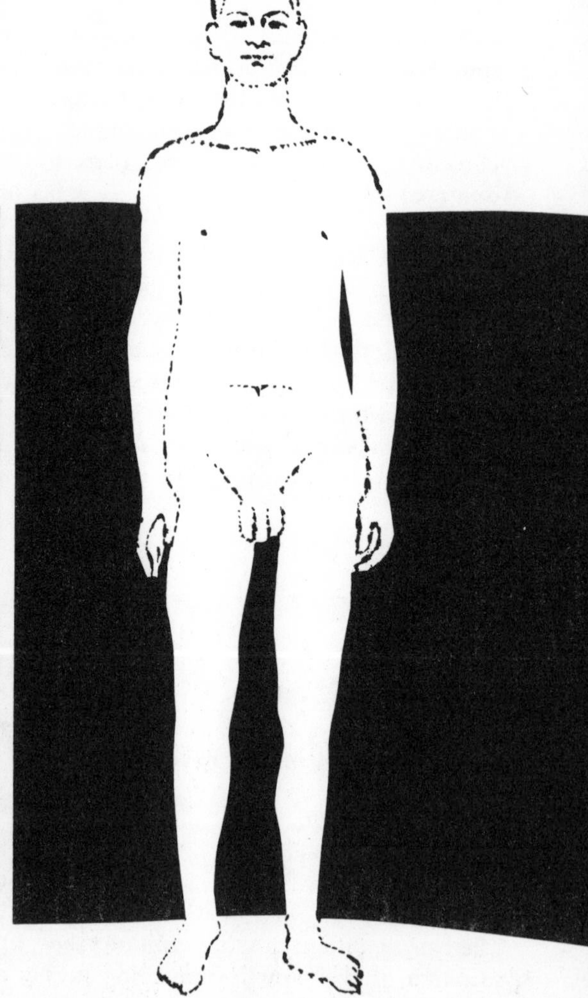

The onset of *acromegaly* occurs gradually after normal maturation of the body has taken place. The bones of the hands, feet and face become abnormally enlarged, and the soft tissues of the nose, ears and cheeks thicken.

**complications**

In neither condition is basic intelligence affected. Giantism may be accomplished by other metabolic disturbances, and the sexual drive may either be lost entirely or abnormally intensified. Acromegaly may be complicated by disturbances in vision, by muscle pains, fatigue, and weakness of sexual impulses. A significant number of adult victims develop diabetic symptoms and heart disorders.

**treatment**

Hyperactivity of the pituitary gland in childhood may respond to certain types of hormone treatment. Since the onset of the condition in adulthood is usually triggered by the development of a tumor, treatment consists of radiation therapy or surgical removal, or a combination of both.

▶ The Endocrine Glands, *The Pituitary Gland,* 1050.

**ACROPHOBIA.** *See* PHOBIAS.

**ACROSCLEROSIS,** a chronic progressive disease involving the hardening of the skin and blood vessels of the hands and sometimes of the ankles. The skin becomes waxy, smooth, leathery, and tight. The face loses its expression, becoming masklike. The individual becomes weak and loses weight. The blood supply to the fingers, toes, ears, and nose is diminished, especially during cold weather. Acrosclerosis is one of the *collagen diseases,* ailments of the connective tissues of the body. The cause is unknown and treatment is rarely satisfactory. *See also* COLLAGEN *and* **medigraphs** RAYNAUD'S DISEASE; SCLERODERMA.

**ACTH,** the abbreviation for *adrenocorticotropic hormone.* ACTH is produced by the *anterior lobe* of the *pituitary gland.* The bloodstream carries the hormone to the *adrenal glands,* situated just above the kidneys. There, ACTH stimulates the *cortex* (outer layer) of the adrenals to produce *corticosterone* and other hormones. If the pituitary does not produce sufficient ACTH, the adrenal cortex will become smaller and its output of hormones will decline.

Unlike some other hormones, ACTH has not yet been synthesized in the laboratory. It is isolated from the pituitary glands of cattle and pigs. Injected into humans, ACTH is used to treat many diseases, including certain allergies and asthma. It has an anti-inflammation action which makes it useful in the treatment of rheumatoid arthritis and rheumatic fever. ACTH is being used experimentally in other illnesses. *See also* ADRENAL GLANDS; ADRENAL GLAND DISORDERS; PITUITARY.

**ACTINOMYCES,** a fungus responsible for causing actinomycosis, a serious disease of pigs and cattle. A related organism causes this disease in humans, but it is rare. *See also* ACTINOMYCOSIS.

**ACTINOMYCIN,** an antibiotic used to treat actinomycosis and other bacterial and fungal infections. One form of actinomycin is used in the management of certain types of cancer. *See also* ANTIBIOTICS.

**ACTINOMYCOSIS,** a fungus infection involving the deep tissues of the skin and mucous membranes, usually of the face, neck, chest and abdomen. It usually affects cattle and hogs but may be transmitted to humans. People working on farms acquire the disease by handling or chewing straw used by infected cattle or by inhaling dust where infected animals are kept. The fungus inhabits the mucous membranes of the mouth, the areas around decayed teeth, and diseased tonsils. The disease begins as a swelling of the jaw, which characteristically has a lumpy feeling. Actinomycosis is sometimes called *lumpy jaw*. The skin turns dark red and abscesses develop. In humans, about half the cases of actinomycosis affect only the face and neck areas. Sometimes, it travels to the chest region and involves the lungs and air passages. It may also affect the abdomen, causing a large internal abscess or one that drains pus outside the body. The most unusual forms of the disease affect the brain, heart valves, or the anus. Cattle and hogs infected with this disease must be destroyed.

In humans, actinomycosis was once almost always fatal, but now can be treated successfully with penicillin or other antibiotics. Treatment also includes x-ray therapy and draining of the abscesses. *See also* FUNGUS.

**ACUPUNCTURE,** an ancient Oriental medical treatment, consisting of inserting long, slender needles into specific points on the body in order to cure disease or relieve pain. Silver, gold, or steel needles, up to 10 inches long, are inserted into one or more of 365 parts of the body, and are twirled rapidly. The points of insertion have been precisely mapped, and Chinese practitioners use anatomical charts showing these points.

**Acupuncture**—Surgeons remove a portion of stomach from a person anesthetized by needle insertion into the outer ear.

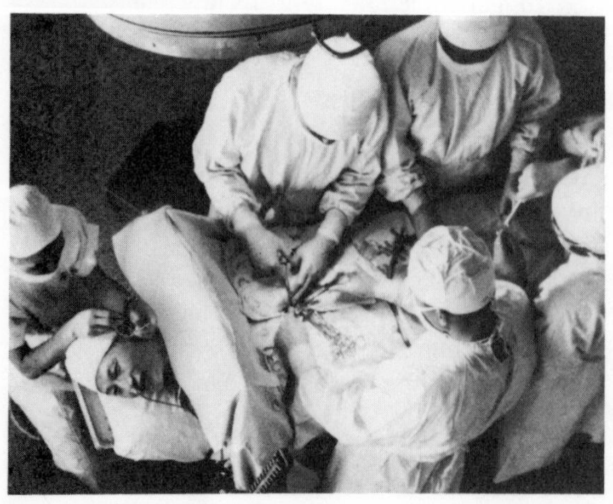

Acupuncture has become well known to Americans in recent years, since the People's Republic of China and the United States entered into normal relations. Acupuncture has begun to be used on an experimental basis by specialists in a few American clinics.

American physicians who have visited Chinese hospitals and observed the use of acupuncture there have reported that it is used successfully in place of anesthesia, even in major surgery.

A satisfactory explanation for the efficacy of acupuncture has not been offered by either Chinese or Western physicians. However, the anesthetic possibilities of acupuncture are being explored. While some observers have contended that hypnotic suggestion is the basis of acupuncture, proponents of the procedure deny this, maintaining that its effects have a purely physiological foundation.

In Chinese practice, a patient is given a sedative and a qualified anesthesiologist stands by, ready to use conventional methods if acupuncture does not work. If it is successful, the patient remains awake during surgery. The surgical procedures themselves—as distinguished from use of needles as an anesthetic—are identical to those of Western hospitals. Observers have reported that surgical patients read, drink fruit juices, or chat with the doctors and nurses during an operation.

Authorities on pain believe that acupuncture somehow sends signals to the brain that compete with or eliminate pain signals that ordinarily would accompany surgery. They also suspect that the psychological component of successful acu-

**Acupuncture,** used in China since 200 B.C. and introduced into Japan in 573 A.D., is a method of treating numerous disorders and of anesthetization that is in standard use in present-day Chinese medicine, and which has been used experimentally in the West. Acupuncture is based on the theory that illnesses of the body are caused by a temporary imbalance of a "life force" (*ch'i*) that controls all bodily processes. Such imbalances can be corrected either by stimulating or reducing the "force" at certain key points in the body. This is done with twirling needles which are inserted at the key points controlling the particular complaint.

According to acupuncture theory, the "life force" flows along "meridians" throughout the body. Over the centuries Chinese physicians have drawn up elaborate maps of these meridians, and indicated 365 key points distributed along these meridians (see diagram, *right*).

Although the theory of a life force flowing in meridians has never been scientifically validated, acupuncture treatment is known to have been beneficial in cases of arthritis.

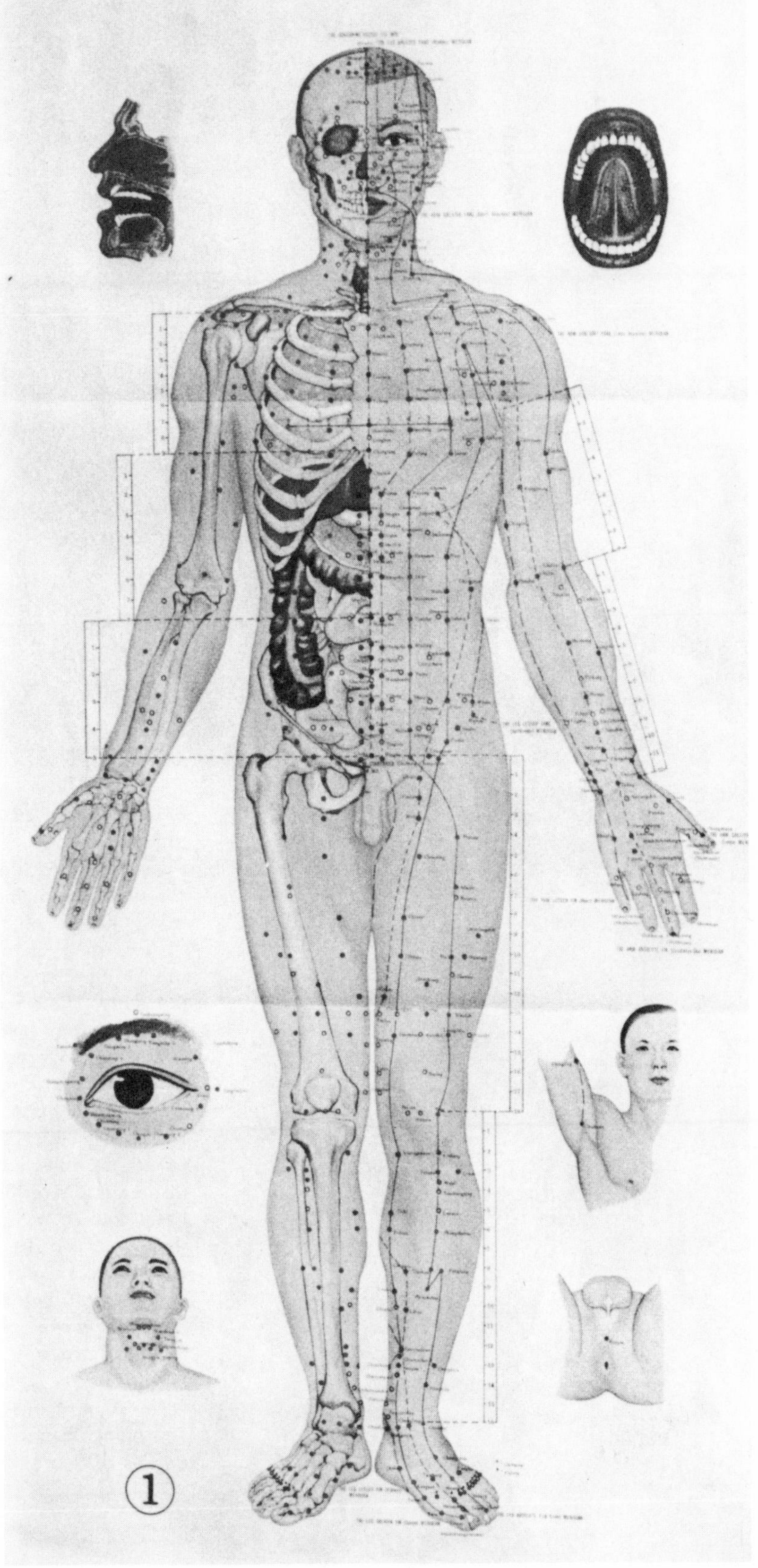

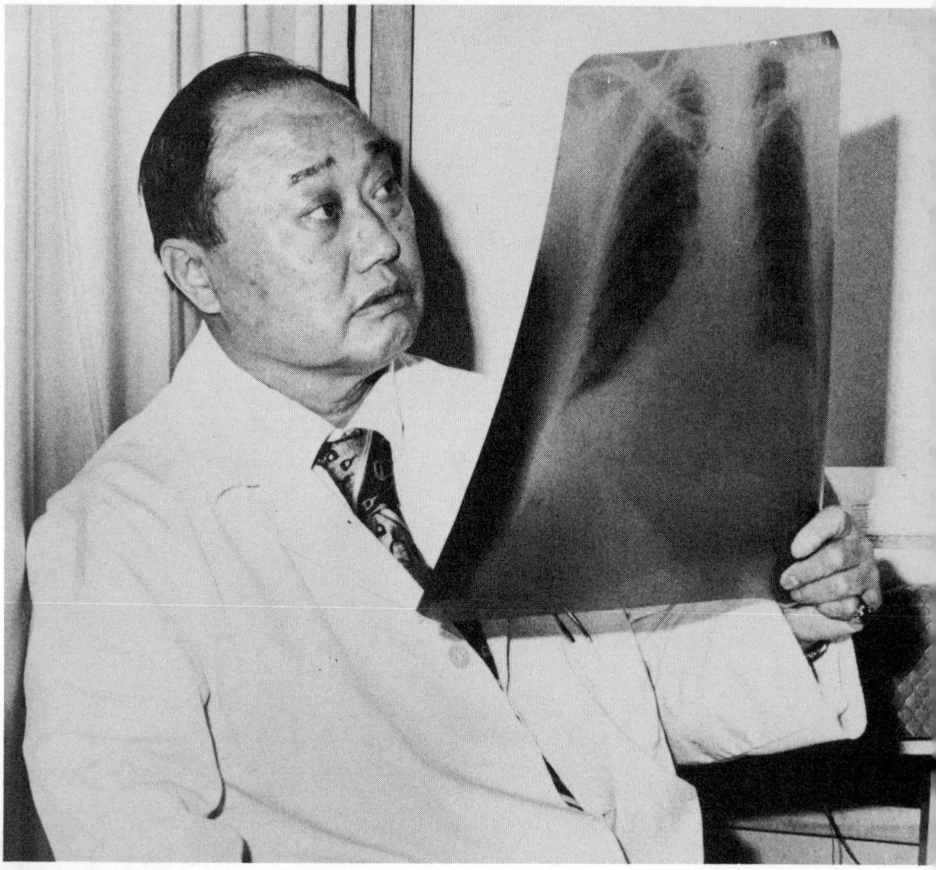

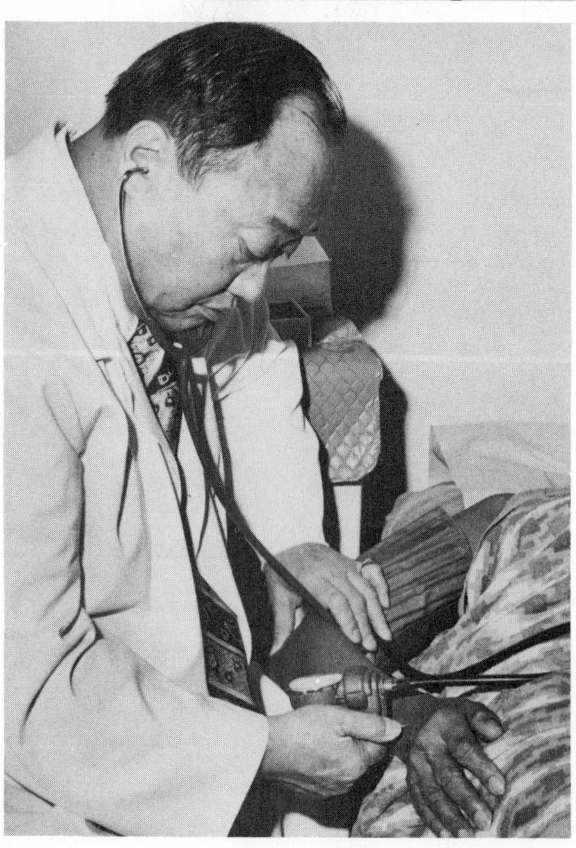

**Before giving acupuncture treatment,** the physician administers a standard medical examination to identify the ailment. *Above,* the doctor examines a chest x-ray. *Left,* he takes the patient's blood pressure.

According to acupuncture theory, there are 14 meridians running lengthwise through the body. These meridians govern all the internal organs and bodily processes. The meridians have no connection with the nervous system or circulatory system. It must be added that these "meridians" have never been seen under a microscope; and there is as yet no objective evidence that they actually exist. Nevertheless, acupuncturists have been known to obtain good results with their empirical treatments in a wide variety of disorders. Whether these results can be properly attributed to the actual treatments or to the power of suggestion is still a matter of controversy among scientists.

The theory states that key points on the various meridians control bodily functions. The points themselves are often far from the organs they are said to govern.

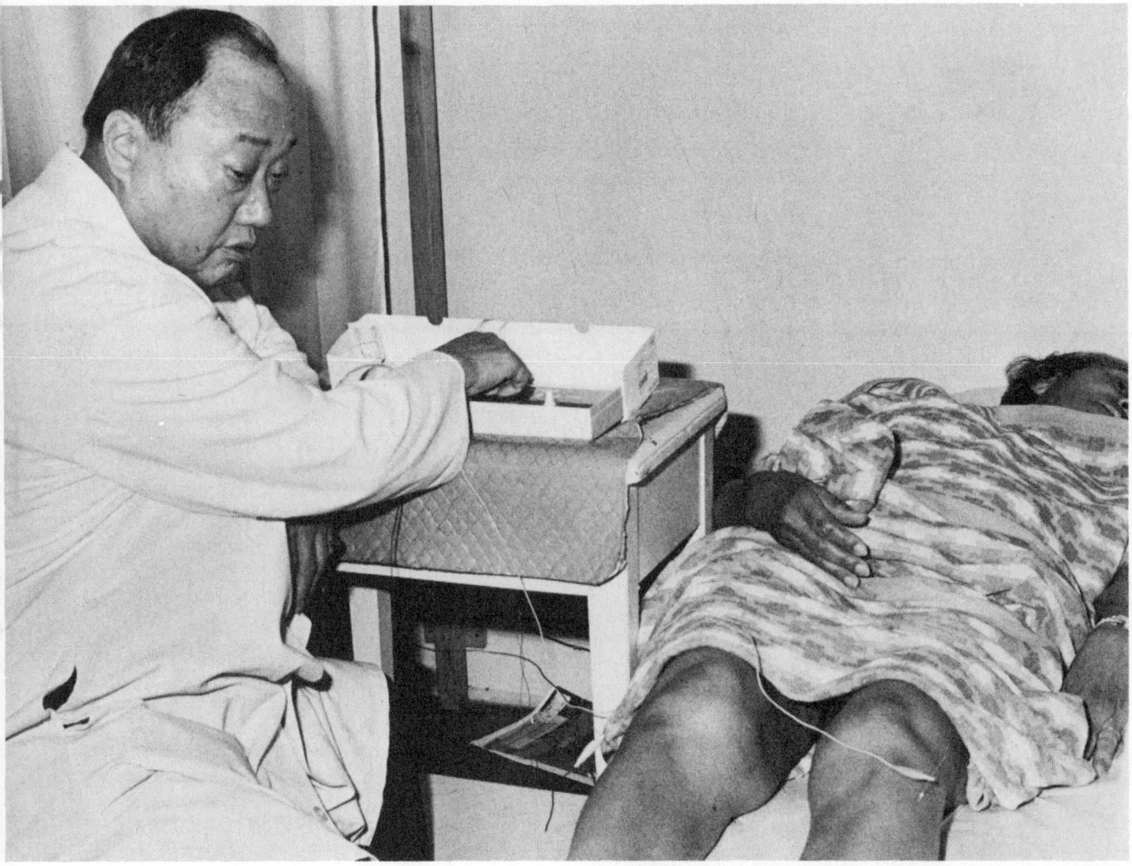

Needles are delicately inserted and carefully twirled at key points on the meridians to treat disorders. In modern acupuncture practice, the needles may be electrically sensitized (*above* and *right*). This patient is being treated for arthritis. A needle is inserted at a key meridian point in her leg.

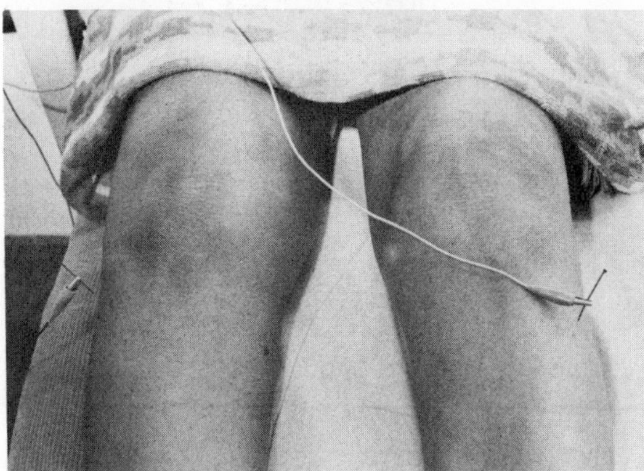

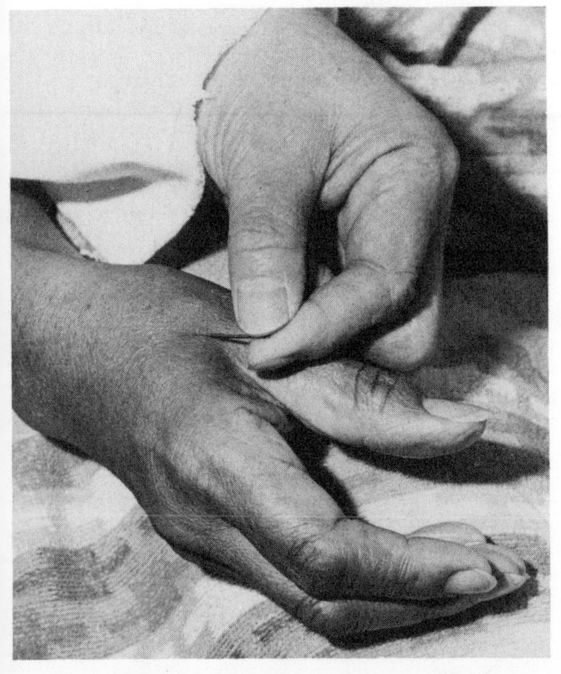

Another needle is inserted and manipulated at a key point in the hand (*left*). This woman showed considerable improvement after this treatment. Acupuncture has been most effective in such disorders as arthritis, neuralgia, headaches, and other metabolic malfunctions. It can neither cure nor prevent diseases caused by germs, and cannot be used to treat cancer.

In recent years, acupuncture has been employed as an effective anesthetic in surgical operations.

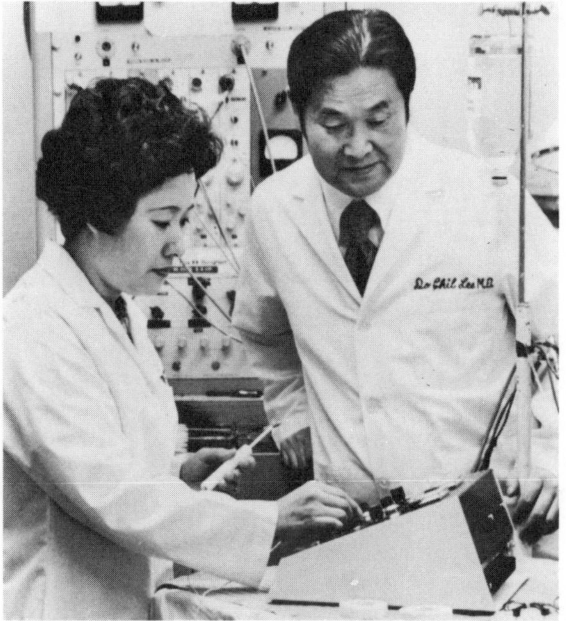

**Acupuncture**—This research team uncovered preliminary evidence in animals that acupuncture works through the autonomic nervous system—the part of the nervous system controlling involuntary functions such as heartbeat and the digestive and respiratory systems. The researchers induced instrument-measurable heart and blood vessel effects in anesthetized dogs with acupuncture. Then they blocked these effects with a drug that specifically interferes with a division of the autonomic nervous system. Their findings provide an explanation for the heretofore unexplained ancient procedure. Since the dogs were anesthetized, hypnosis or psychosomatic suggestion as the basis of acupuncture is well disputed.

puncture is strong, and that the procedure works most effectively with persons who are generally friendly, cooperative, helpful, and strong believers in the principles of a religious or political system. Possibly a degree of self-hypnosis in controlling pain is significant.

Although acupuncture has received public attention primarily because of its use as an anesthetic, Chinese physicians report that it is effective in the treatment of a variety of ailments, including headache, arthritis, heart diseases, and chest disorders. *See also* ANESTHESIA.

RESEARCH REPORT

### ACUPUNCTURE RESULTS ACHIEVED THROUGH AUTONOMIC NERVOUS SYSTEM

Studies by a team of anesthesiologists at the MEDICAL COLLEGE OF OHIO indicate that *acupuncture* achieves its effects primarily through the body's *autonomic nervous system* rather than through hypnosis or autosuggestion.

On the assumption that unconscious animals would be impervious to psychological influences, the researchers began their tests by anesthetizing dogs with *halothane* and used acupuncture techniques which induced instrument-measurable cardiovascular changes in their subjects. These responses were then blocked by a drug whose action specifically interferes with a part of the autonomic nervous system.

The researchers observed that acupuncture corrected minor naturally-occurring cardiovascular aberrations such as irregular heartbeat and pulse variations. These results led to the conclusion that the effect of acupuncture was mediated through the autonomic nervous system, since the drug *atropin* produces similar results through the same body mechanism.

Similarly, the effects of *epinephrine* (*adrenalin*) in reversing cardiac arrest and increasing cardiac output were duplicated in the anesthetized animals by using acupuncture. Adrenalin stimulates the sympathetic division of the autonomic nervous system.

As a further check, the investigators ran experiments with the anesthetic *propranolol* which specifically blocks certain chemical secretions of the sympathetic nervous system. In these tests, the propranolol blocked the cardiovascular effects of the acupuncture procedures which would ordinarily stimulate certain elements of the sympathetic nervous system.

The acupuncture point used to increase cardiac output in the anesthetized animals is known as Jen-Chung or GO-26 and is located at the medium vertical groove of the upper lip. Cardiac arrest was reversed at an acupuncture point (ST-9) in the neck near the larynx. Normal pulse was restored through a point (LI-5) equivalent to the interior side of the wrist joint in humans. NIH515

**ACUTE,** a medical term signifying the abrupt onset of an ailment. The opposite term is *chronic*—signifying the prolonged duration of a disorder, usually at a less intense level. The acute phase of any disease, though brief, may be severe, requiring immediate and possibly emergency attention and treatment.

**ADAM'S APPLE,** a projection of the thyroid cartilage at the front of the throat, enclosing and protecting the two vocal cords. The Adam's apple actually consists of the left and right thyroid cartilages, meeting at a right angle and making the easily noticed projection that sometimes appears to ride up and down at the knot of a man's necktie. It is more prominent in men than in women, because the angle in a man's Adam's apple is sharper and there is usually less fat in the neck. The picturesque name derives from the Biblical first man and the forbidden fruit he ate. *See also* LARYNX.

**ADAPTATION,** the adjustment of an organism, whether a plant, animal or man, to its environment. Adaptation also refers to the ability of a part of the body to adjust. For example, the pupil of the eye automatically adapts itself to the amount of light striking it. It does this quickly, so that within a few seconds, a person going from a brightly lit area to semi-darkness can see satisfactorily. Humans adapt well, so that they can survive in cold or hot climates, in rainy or dry seasons, and under either sparsely populated or crowded conditions. They can also adapt to stress. The human organs and glandular system enable people to live and work under different circumstances and to relax when the stress conditions are removed. An entire species, human or animal, also may adapt slowly to radically changed circumstances through the process of evolution.

▶ Stress Without Distress, *Historic Development,* 2760; *Syntoxic and Catatoxic Responses,* 2762.

**ADDICTION,** physiological or psychological dependence on a substance, such as alcohol or heroin, and a tendency to require increasing amounts of the substance. Another evidence of addiction is the occurrence of physical or psychological *withdrawal symptoms* if the substance is suddenly taken away. These symptoms may include severe pain, nausea, cramps, hallucinations and violent headaches. They also may be milder, such as irritability, insomnia, restlessness during the day, and a desire for the substance so strong that the victim carries out normal activities with difficulty.

A person can become addicted to legally prescribed medication as well as to such illegal drugs as heroin or cocaine. Doctors limit the number of times prescriptions for certain medications can be refilled to protect their patients from addiction. However, tranquilizers, sedatives, and barbiturates are used illicitly by many people who may become dependent on them without realizing what is happening. Users of sleeping pills know that over a long time, they require higher doses to achieve sleep.

An unfortunate trend over the past decade has been the indiscriminate prescribing of certain drugs by some doctors. Rather than delve further to uncover treatable causes of a patient's fatigue, anxiety or tension, they simply write a prescription for an amphetamine or a tranquilizer. By far, women are the chief recipients of this type of treatment, and alarming numbers of them are becoming addicted to their medications.

Psychological addiction, or *dependence,* is a problem for smokers. Long-term smokers know how difficult it is to stop, or even to taper off. The combination of a strong habit and physical and psychological dependence creates difficulties for anyone who stops smoking. Weeks or months may pass before a former smoker can feel comfortable and adjust to a nonsmoking life. Even then, if he returns to smoking for only a day or two, he usually is just as dependent again as though he had never stopped. *See also* ALCOHOL; DRUG ABUSE; DRUG WITHDRAWAL; MORPHINE; OPIUM AND OPIATES; TOBACCO *and* **medigraphs** ALCOHOLISM; AMPHETAMINE ABUSE; BARBITURATE ABUSE; COCAINE ABUSE; HEROIN ABUSE.

# ADDICTION'S VICIOUS CIRCLE

**Barbiturates bring sleep, opiates kill pain. But like other mood-changing drugs they carry the risk of addiction, where body and personality are ruined by the need for an ever larger dose.**

THE ABUSE OF DRUGS CONSTITUTES a major present-day problem. Drugs, and in particular alcohol, have been used as a source of pleasure as far back in history as records go. But in modern society, too, there are social and cultural pressures that encourage the taking of drugs, whether it be the drinking of alcohol or the smoking of cigarettes. It is when this indulgence becomes harmful both to society and the individual that it is condemned.

The term *drug addiction* is now, strictly speaking, obsolete. In the past this term was used to describe the type of addiction found with drugs such as heroin.

The danger does not lie in the initial effects, but in the fact that these drugs produce both physical and psychological dependence. In *physical dependence* the drug produces changes in the body's functioning; not only do unpleasant physical symptoms occur when the drug is withdrawn, but the body habituates itself to the drug's effects and larger and larger doses are required. This phenomenon is known as *tolerance. Psychological dependence* refers to the inability of addicts to face life and its problems without drugs. As a result of these various factors, the addict is forced to continue to take drugs because of being unable to face the mental and physical torture which would follow giving them up.

These three features—physical and psychological dependence and the development of tolerance—were considered to be the hallmark of the addictive drugs. A distinction was made between drugs of this type—commonly called *hard* drugs—and *soft* drugs such as the amphetamines and barbiturates, which were only regarded as habit forming and were widely prescribed. This distinction between hard and soft drugs is an unfortunate one, as it has tended to minimize the dangers of the supposedly soft drugs. Psychological dependence, which is a feature of these drugs, is now recognized as the most important factor in drug dependence.

The World Health Organization recommended that the term *drug dependence* should replace that of drug addiction. The characteristics of this dependence, whether physical or psychological, or both, will vary with the drug that is being used.

### THE MAIN ADDICTIVES

Although there are some individuals who can become psychologically dependent on substances which do not produce physical reactions, there are certain main groups of drugs which are generally recognized as producing dependency problems. These are the opiates, alcohol and the barbiturates, the amphetamines and cocaine, the hallucinogens, and cannabis.

Opium, the traditional drug of the East, has its more potent but pharmacologically similar equivalents in the West. Heroin and morphine are the best-known members of this group. Taken by mouth, or more commonly by injection into a vein, these drugs—the opiates—produce in the user a sense of extreme well-being and relaxation. They find their main medical use in the relief of pain and, up until about 1960, practically all individuals who were dependent on these drugs had either been introduced to them as part of medical treatment or had ready access to them through their work. Doctors and nurses, for instance, formed quite a high proportion of such addicts. In recent years there has been an alarming increase in the number of young people using these drugs, obtained illicitly in the first place. Because of the lack of care taken when injecting themselves, blood infections and jaundice are common. In the United States today, the form most readily available and cheapest is brown heroin from Mexico. By the time it reaches users, it is only two to ten percent pure since it is usually diluted by sellers.

Because it does not conform to the standard pattern of addiction seen with the opiates, the problem of alcohol (and, to a lesser extent, barbiturate) dependency has tended to be considered as something quite different from other forms of drug dependency. One point of difference is that alcohol is in common social usage, as to a lesser extent are the barbiturates in the form of sleeping tablets.

Alcohol has the effect of reducing tension while increasing confidence, particularly in social situations. Barbiturates also reduce feelings of tension and anxiety but pro-

**Two different addictions require quite dissimilar equipment. The addict at left needs only a bottle of some kind of alcoholic drink. More complex paraphernalia (*right*) is needed for the heroin addict—especially a tourniquet to make the vein stand out and a syringe to make the injection.**

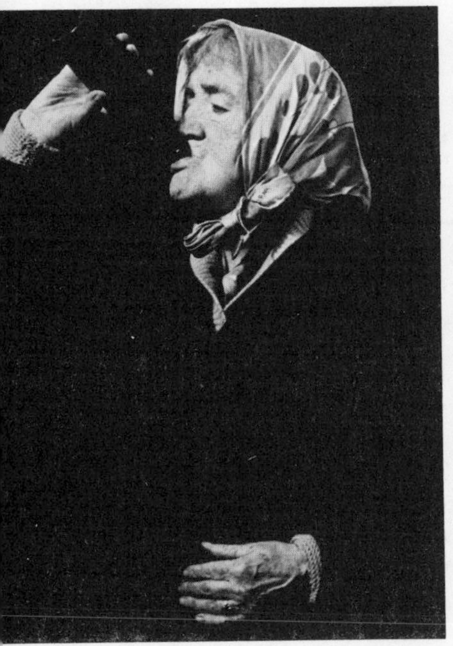

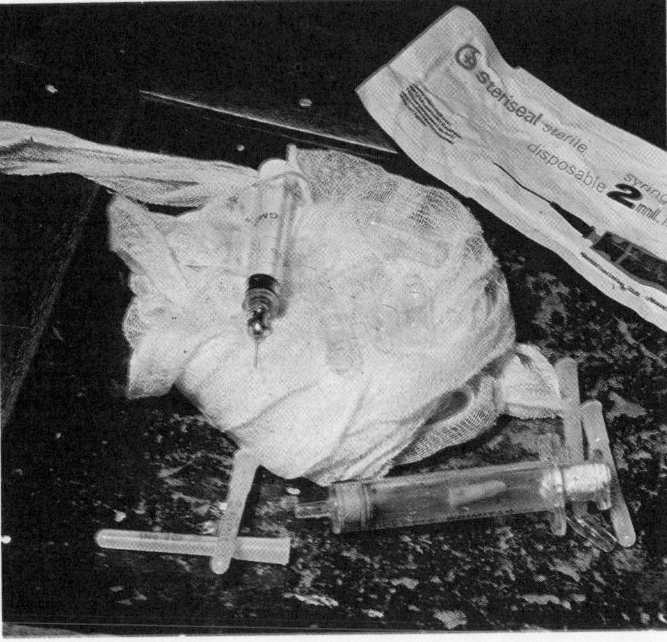

duce as well a hypnotic effect. Overindulgence in either alcohol or barbiturates produces unsteadiness of gait and slurring of speech. Both lower inhibitions and impair judgment and someone under their influence, no longer governed by customary restraint, is likely to say and do things he would not say and do normally.

Because alcohol is in common social use and the amount of alcohol taken varies so widely from person to person, alcoholism is difficult to define. The term is probably best reserved for those whose dependence on alcohol has reached such a degree that they either show noticeable physical or mental disturbance or are unable to maintain their normal social relationships.

Barbiturate dependency possibly occupies for women the position that alcoholism does for men. Studies have revealed that of American women not holding jobs outside the home, 48 percent were using or had used a mood-altering drug obtained with legitimate prescription. Though some were for stimulating amphetamines, most were for the antianxiety drugs such as barbiturates and tranquilizers. Although tolerance to barbiturates develops, the margin between the dose tolerated and a lethal dose is small. This sometimes leads to the deaths of barbiturate-dependent individuals by taking an accidental overdose.

Substances similar to the present-day amphetamines were used by the Chinese. However, these drugs have only been produced on a commercial scale since the 1930s, and the misuse of amphetamines has only become a social problem more recently still. One effect of amphetamines is to reduce appetite, so they used to be prescribed as diet pills. Tolerance would develop, more amphetamines would have to be taken and a mental illness very similar to paranoid schizophrenia was sometimes the result.

For the younger age group amphetamines produce just those effects which are much sought after by teenagers—increased alertness, confidence and talkativeness. The shy, inhibited, self-conscious teenager is able to talk and dance all night. When the effect wears off the teenager feels irritable and depressed, but taking more tablets relieves these symptoms. Characteristically, they are taken first over weekends for "kicks," then perhaps during the week as well, and finally the individual cannot do without them and has to take them all the time. Some may go on to inject the drug, or graduate to the opiates. However, only a small proportion of those who start taking amphetamines progress to a severe amphetamine-dependent state.

Cocaine stimulates the central nervous system and produces a feeling of excitement and well-being. In Bolivia and Peru the peasants still rely on this addictive drug to make their hard lives tolerable.

The hallucinogens are drugs which can produce bizarre perceptual disturbances, mainly of sound and vision. These drugs are generally called by the letters of the chemical compounds they are made from; lysergic acid diethylamide, for example, is more commonly known as LSD. This very powerful drug often produces disorientation in both time and space, plus radical changes of mood, and for these reasons is considered dangerous.

Cannabis—commonly known as marijuana or hashish—is by international agreement classified as a dependency-producing drug, although the evidence for this is inconclusive. Its main effects are to produce a feeling of excitement and to bring about changes in the appreciation of time and space, but there is considerable individual variation. Much controversy centers around the possible effects of marijuana and how likely its use is to lead to the hard drugs. One report has suggested that marijuana cigarettes may contain higher concentrations of cancer-causing agents than tobacco cigarettes. A 1976 survey revealed that in the course of a year more than half of all 23-year-old males smoked some marijuana. The nationwide trend has been toward a considerable reduction in penalties for possession of this "soft" drug. In certain states, possession of small amounts has been decriminalized with the penalty now usually only a small fine.

As with all drugs, social and cultural factors are probably of as much importance as the personality of the individual in determining who does and who does not take the drug. Conformity to the standards of a group, a desire to flout parents and authority, belief in a drug's mystic properties and its powers to widen the range of experience—all are probably factors in drug-taking.

Apart from its tragic effects on the addict, the taking of all the main types of drugs may have serious social consequences. With the opiates, although it is possible to be dependent on them for long periods without showing evidence of physical and social deterioration, such cases are in fact the exception. The difficulties of obtaining regular supplies of his drug dominate the opiate addict's outlook on life. General attention to physical health and dress is neglected and any means, legitimate or illegitimate, are taken to ensure a supply of the drug.

Alcoholism is the largest drug problem in the United States today. The number of alcoholics in the country is estimated to range from six to 14 million. Drinking tends to increase as people move up the socioeconomic scale—surveys show that about 80 percent of upper class people and 70 percent in the middle class drink, but only 48 percent of those in the lower socioeconomic group drink. More men drink than women and men generally drink three times as much as women. But women are catching up—more of them drink and women are drinking greater amounts. Another significant trend is to earlier and heavy drinking in adolescence. It has been estimated that 1.3 million Americans between 12 and 17 years of age have a serious drinking problem.

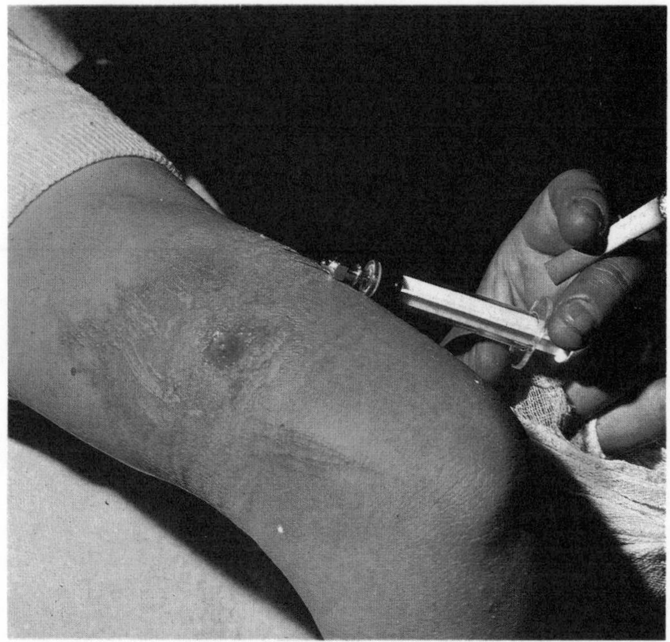

**Because heroin addicts often are careless about cleanliness when injecting themselves, infections are common among them. Another problem is jaundice, which frequently results from using a contaminated needle.**

The impaired perception produced by alcohol is well known; even small amounts interfere with coordination and judgment. Cannabis impairs time perception and, like alcohol, can reduce the capacity to drive an automobile or other vehicle.

The increased assertiveness and self-confidence produced by amphetamines have often led to serious social consequences. Taking and driving away cars, breaking and entering are typical examples of antisocial behavior under their influence.

Perhaps more serious have been the distorted perceptions of those on the hallucinogens, who are recorded as having jumped out of windows believing they could fly or rushed out into the streets believing in their divine power to stop traffic. There are, as well, acts of homicide recorded in connection with the abuse of LSD.

Because of the variety of drugs involved in dependency and the social and cultural problems it raises, treatment has many different facets. Dependency can occur in all sorts and all conditions of persons, and the problems presented and the treatment required will be correspondingly different.

### WITHDRAWAL OF DRUGS

The original medical approach was to attempt withdrawal of the drug, either directly or by substituting some less harmful drug. With the opiates this is almost always done on an inpatient basis. The relapse rate is high, patients usually discharging themselves soon after the drug has been withdrawn. In this case there is an added danger that the individual will return to the dose of drug being taken before entering the hospital and, because tolerance has decreased, may accidentally become overdosed. With individuals using cocaine or the amphetamines, however, the aim of treatment must be to withdraw the drug because of the risk of mental deterioration.

Methadone, given to drug users as a substitute for opiates, is in itself addictive. However, it is inexpensive and the addict can remain on it without having to resort to crime to pay for the habit. It is not the answer it was once hoped to be and many addicts fail to stay in methadone treatment. But ten years of methadone programs have reached larger numbers of addicts than other programs, and have significantly reduced heroin use.

Attempts can also be made to make the taking of the drug an unpleasant event rather than a pleasant event. *Antabuse* is employed for this purpose in the treatment of alcoholism, its effect being to produce nausea and vomiting in the patient when he takes a drink. The patient, it is hoped, learns to associate alcohol with feeling sick and therefore stops drinking.

However, it is not enough merely to withdraw the drug. Rehabilitation aims not only to re-educate the individual to live without drugs but also to help the person to live a normal social life. This means help in overcoming any particular personal difficulty that might be making a person cling to drugs, but, above all, it means providing emotional support. One organization which aims to do this is Alcoholics Anonymous. Regular evening meetings are held which provide encouragement and reassurance for those with an alcohol problem. Unfortunately, only a minority of the patients who are encouraged to join do so. There are many extensive organizations for the rehabilitation of those with drug problems, such as Phoenix Houses, run for and by drug addicts, where patients may spend several years. In many of these schemes the cured addict may help in the treatment of new addicts.

Drug dependency is essentially a chronic relapsing condition and, therefore, it is usually not practical to speak in terms of absolute cure. Those who are most likely to remain permanently off drugs are those with a previously stable personality. The young amphetamine user, too, who is only using drugs as a means of solving adolescent problems, has a fairly good chance of recovering. For the majority, however, the most realistic goal of treatment is to aim at helping a damaged and handicapped individual to adjust to his or her environment.

In all countries where drug dependency has been a serious problem, attempts to limit the spread of drugs have usually involved controlling their source and means of supply. Education as a means of control appears unlikely to be very effective. The campaign to stop people smoking exemplifies this; people take drugs for emotional reasons and the knowledge of future hazards does not seem to be a practical deterrent. Public opinion is probably a very important instrument of control but, as the debate on marijuana shows, public opinion is rarely unanimous.

Legal control in some countries has attempted to impose a total ban on the manufacture, prescription and sale of certain drugs. Both the United States and Sweden impose such controls but in both countries severe drug-dependency problems still exist. In Great Britain certain drugs, such as heroin, have been available only from prescribed sources. However, a small number of medical practitioners have been found to be prescribing very large quantities of drugs, and the system of licensing has therefore been adopted.

Only Japan has overcome a serious drug problem. In 1954 there were reported to be 1,000,000 individuals misusing amphetamines. By a combination of legislation, strong police methods, the provision of a large number of hospital beds for treatment and by educating the public, the problem was reduced to negligible proportions. This comprehensive approach, however, only succeeded because public opinion was strongly and unitedly behind it.

A grave danger facing every addict is overdose. Lifesaving treatment must be based on the specific drug and the amount taken. Below, urine from a comatose person is being analyzed by a gas chromatograph. A technician monitors the results as the instrument makes the identification.

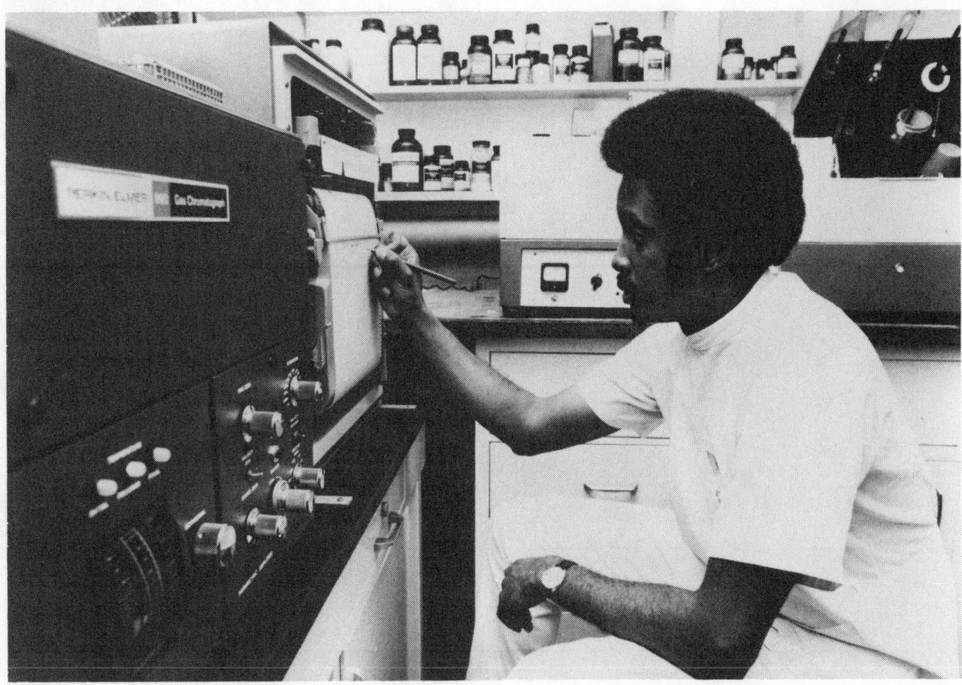

## **Addison's Disease** (Underactivity of the Adrenal Cortex)

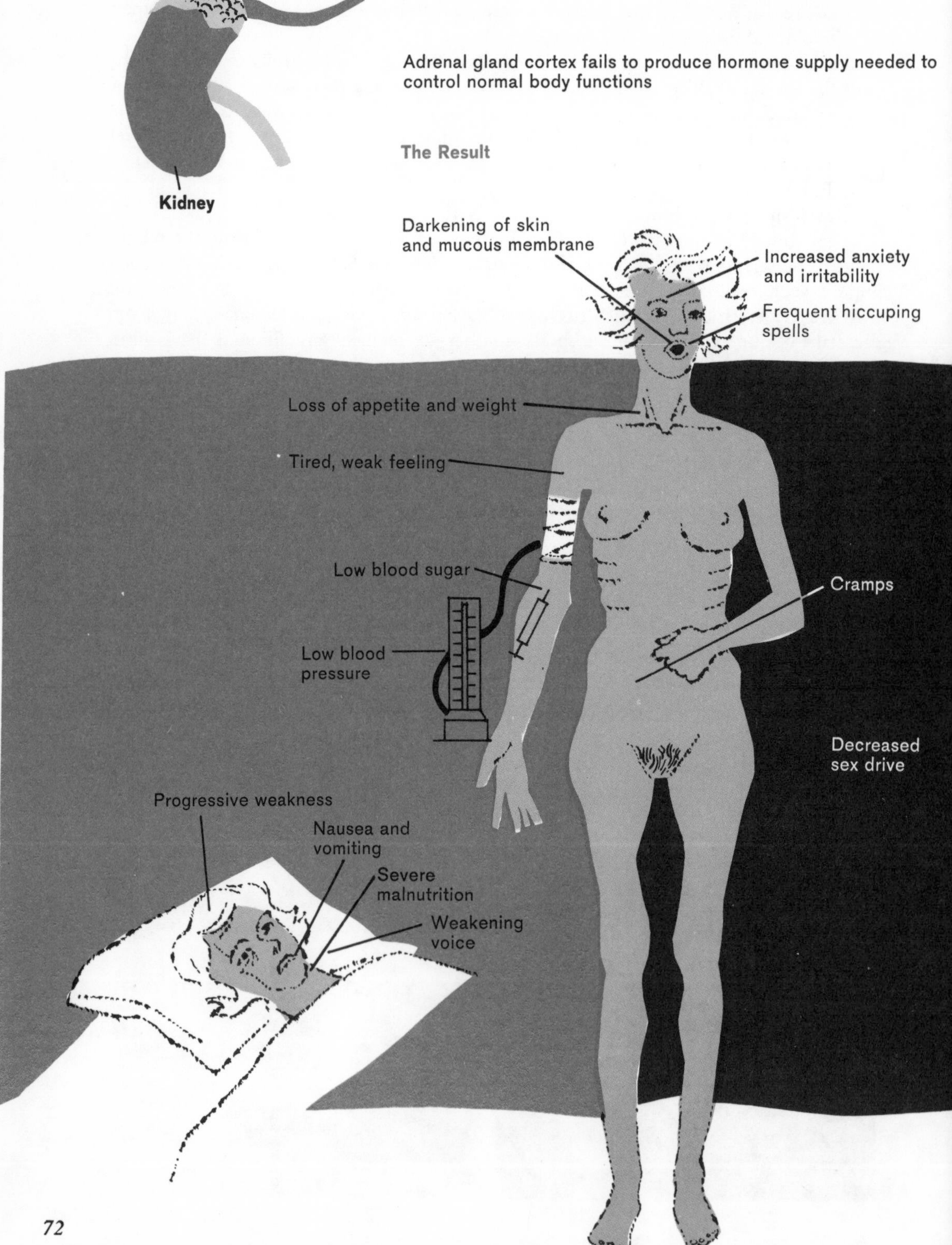

# ADDISON'S DISEASE

FIRST DESCRIBED in 1849 by the London doctor whose name it bears, Addison's disease is a hormonal disorder connected with underactivity (hypofunction) of the *adrenal cortex.*

### causes

The underlying cause for the insufficiency of adrenocortical hormone production in many cases is not yet clear. Tuberculosis of the adrenals, or the development of a tumor, either of which can bring about glandular malfunction, is the explanation in some instances. Although the disorder can occur at any age, it is most commonly encountered during the middle years.

### symptoms

Characteristics of the disease were accurately described by Dr. Addison over a century ago: "anemia, general languor or debility, remarkable feebleness of the heart's action, irritability of the stomach, and a peculiar change of color of the skin." Since the adrenal cortex secretes numerous hormones essential to well-being, hypofunction results in this wide variety of symptoms. Onset of the disease is likely to be insidious, but it expresses itself in the obvious change of skin pigmentation. Weakness and lack of energy resulting from metabolic aberration, deficiency of muscular function, and reduction of cardiac output are chronic symptoms. Weight loss and dehydration may also occur, usually the result of nausea and vomiting. Mental and emotional instability are concomitants of the basic disturbances of body processes.

### complications

Because of the reduced adrenal output, resistance to infection is low and the ability to withstand stress of any kind is markedly impaired. A crisis condition can be precipitated by any acute infection, by surgery, or by excessive sweating leading to serious salt loss.

### treatment

Addison's disease is a chronic condition which can be controlled but not cured. With the administration of various cortisone compounds—either orally or by injection—symptoms are held at a minimum and persons are able to lead comparatively normal lives. This replacement therapy, which is permanent, is often controlled by the patient, who evaluates his own doses in amounts that are therapeutic at the same time that they keep pernicious side effects in check. Patients are usually advised about such matters as diet, salt intake, permissible exercise, and the avoidance of secondary infection and emotional stress.

▶ The Endocrine Glands, *The Pituitary Gland,* 1050.

**ADDUCTOR,** a muscle that draws a portion of the body toward the median line. Fingers, toes, thighs, hips and other areas and portions of the body have both *abductor* and *adductor* muscles, making movement toward or away from the body center quick and easy. *See also* ABDUCTOR; MUSCLE *and* **medigraph** SPRAINS AND STRAINS.

**ADENITIS,** inflammation of a gland. The term is usually applied to the lymph glands, when the condition is more precisely known as *lymphadenitis.* The inflammation and enlargement of the gland usually signify an infection. Since the function of the lymphatic system is to act as a barrier against the spread of infection, the lymph nodes themselves become enlarged and inflamed as microorganisms accumulate.

**ADENOCARCINOMA,** a malignant tumor originating from the glands or from

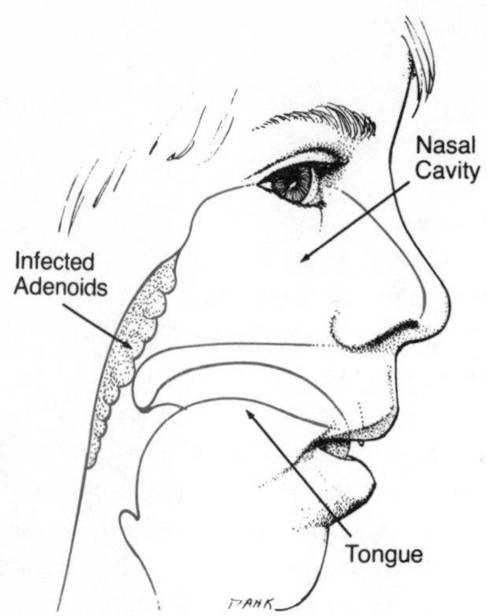


**Adenoids**—When the lymphoid tissues in the back of the throat become infected and enlarged, they interfere with nasal breathing. They can also cause frequent colds and infections in the middle ear which may result in hearing problems.

the lining (*epithelium*) of the body cavities or surfaces. *See also* ADENOMA; CANCER; MALIGNANCY; NEOPLASM.

**ADENOIDS,** a mass of lymphatic tissue in the throat and back of the nose; also called *pharyngeal tonsils*. While this tissue, like all lymphatic tissue, ordinarily serves to collect infectious microorganisms and enable the body to dispose of them, the adenoids, like the tonsils, often become enlarged and infected themselves. In such cases, the doctor may decide that they should be removed as soon as the infection clears up and the tissues resume their normal size and condition. Enlarged adenoids can also block the *Eustachian tubes* (which connect the middle ear with the back of the throat), resulting in pain in the ears and a sense of pressure. Enlarged adenoids may cause a further infection in the middle ear, and occasionally interfere with normal hearing. *Adenoiditis* (inflamed adenoids) is rarely a serious ailment, but it should never be ignored. The adenoids grow until a child is five or six years old. They then diminish slowly, almost disappearing at about the end of adolescence.

A child with infected and inflamed adenoids may have a fever, feel sick, cough, and have trouble breathing. If the condition is chronic, he will catch cold frequently. Also, a chronically adenoidal child will breathe through his mouth. His face takes on a characteristic appearance: the mouth open, the lips turned downward, and the eyes drooping and appearing dull. Formerly, such children often were considered dull or stupid, because of their appearance and because they could not hear well. Of course, adenoiditis has nothing to do with intelligence.

Surgical removal of the adenoids is a simple procedure. The tonsils may be removed at the same time, though this should only be done if they too have been chronically inflamed and infected. An adenoidectomy usually requires a hospital stay of one or two days.

**ADENOMA,** a benign tumor composed of glandular tissue. An adenoma may occur anywhere in the body. Although it is benign, it may grow so large as to interfere with the normal functioning of a body organ. Any growth should be called to the attention of a physician. An adenoma, even an enormous one, can be removed surgically without complications.

## ADENOMA, BRONCHIAL

BRONCHIAL ADENOMA IS A BENIGN tumor occurring in one of the bronchial tubes leading directly into the lungs. Because of the slow growth of such tumors and the symptoms they produce, they may be mistaken for other lung disorders. Bronchial adenomas are relatively rare.

## Bronchial Adenoma

Frequently obstructs air passage and results in partial collapse of lung
Tumor (usually benign)

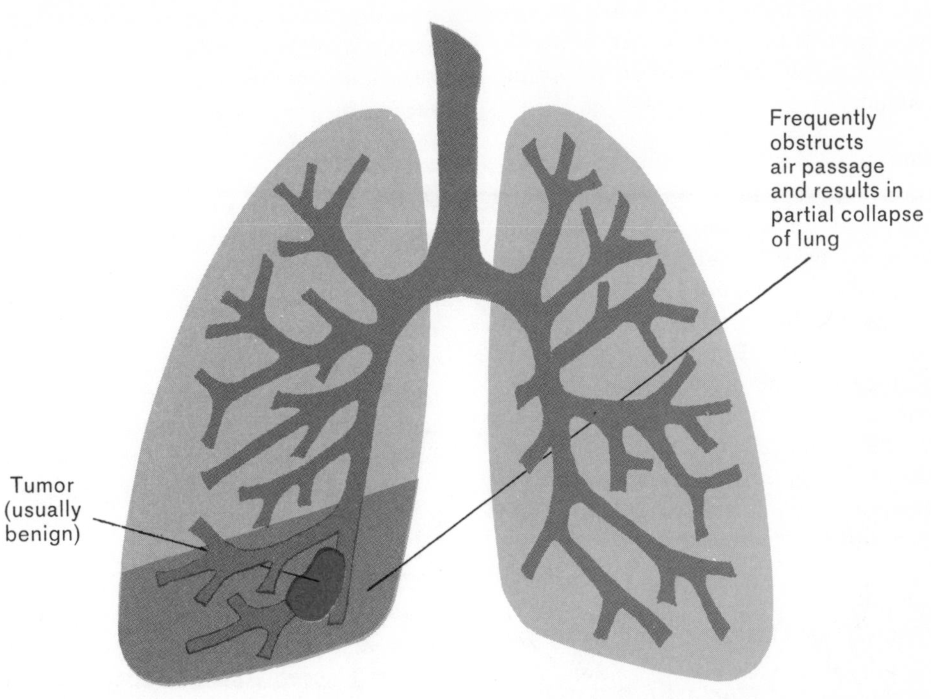

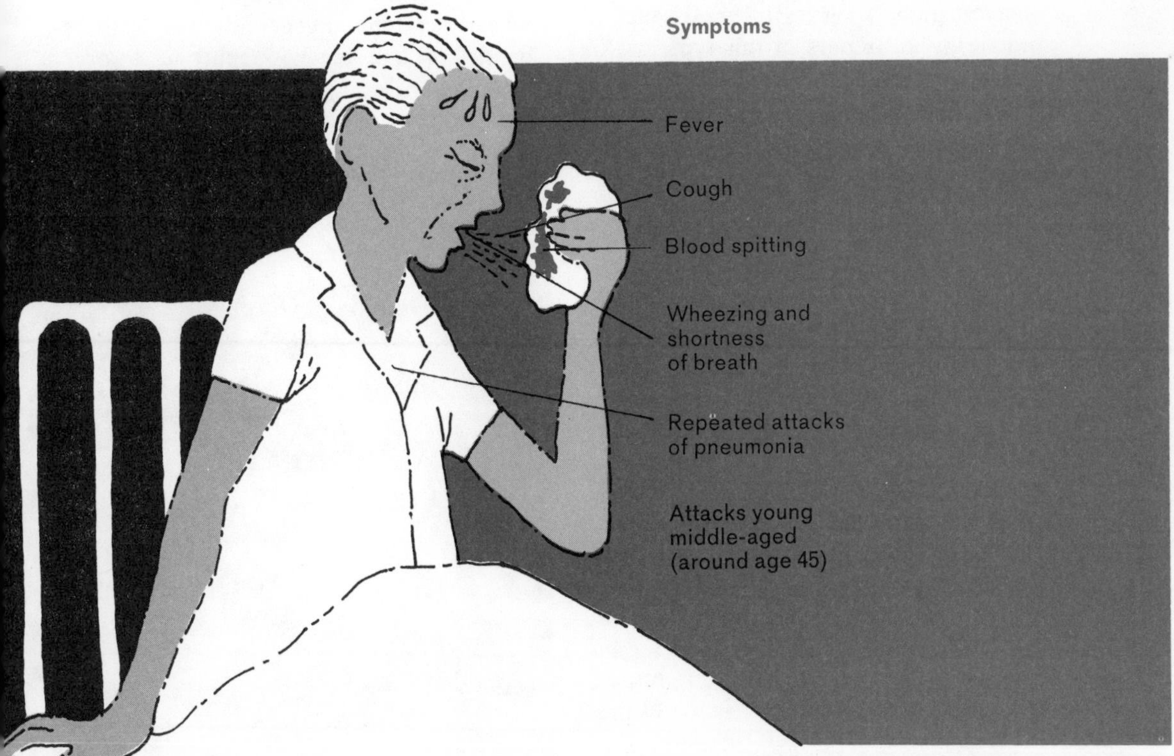

Symptoms
Fever
Cough
Blood spitting
Wheezing and shortness of breath
Repeated attacks of pneumonia
Attacks young middle-aged (around age 45)

**causes**

The cause is unknown, but when the condition is present, it can be aggravated by smoking or by the inhalation of various pollutants in the environment.

**symptoms**

Wheezing, shortness of breath, chest pains, and predisposition to pneumonia are characteristic manifestations. When the growth is large enough it may cause pressure on surrounding tissues or obstruct air flow. Repeated episodes of coughing and spitting up blood may also occur. In some cases, however, symptoms may be completely absent and the presence of the tumor may come to a doctor's attention as the result of a chest x-ray taken during a routine checkup.

**treatment**

Bronchial adenomas are removed by surgery after diagnosis based on x-ray, bronchoscopy and biopsy. Early surgical removal combined in some instances with chemotherapy is successful treatment for practically all tumors of this type.

**ADHESIECTOMY,** the medical term for surgical removal of *adhesions*. *See also* ADHESION.

**ADHESION,** the joining of two body surfaces that are normally separate. The term also refers to the fibrous band that connects the surfaces. Scar tissue following abdominal surgery sometimes causes adhesions to form. Adhesions are usually painless and do not cause difficulty, but sometimes they can cause an obstruction and interfere with the functioning of one or more organs. Since the formation of fibrous scars is a normal biological process, it cannot be entirely prevented by surgical procedure. Surgeons hold adhesions to a minimum by handling internal organs gently, carefully removing all blood from the body cavity, and using warm moist sponges. If adhesions become painful or interfere with normal body functions, further surgery will be necessary to remove them. *See also* SURGERY *and* **medigraph** INTESTINAL OBSTRUCTION.

**ADIPOSIS,** an excessive deposit of fat, usually caused by overeating but sometimes by a physical disorder. The accumulation may be generalized throughout the body, or it may be concentrated in one or more local areas. *Dercum's disease* or *adiposis dolorosa,* is a pathological condition in which fatty masses accumulate under the skin. *Adiposis cerebralis* is generalized fatness caused by a disorder of the pituitary gland. *See also* OBESITY; TUMOR.

**ADJUSTMENT PROBLEMS of the school-age child.** The child in his early school years seems to be living on a calm plateau. The remarkably fast growth, the toilet training, learning to talk, and all the other "civilizing" processes of infancy and early childhood years are completed. The storms and the new spurt of emotional and physical growth of adolescence seem far away. When children first go to

**Adjustment Problems** of the school-age child—Making all kinds of new friends is one of the happy things about going to school. These first-graders are obviously delighted with each other.

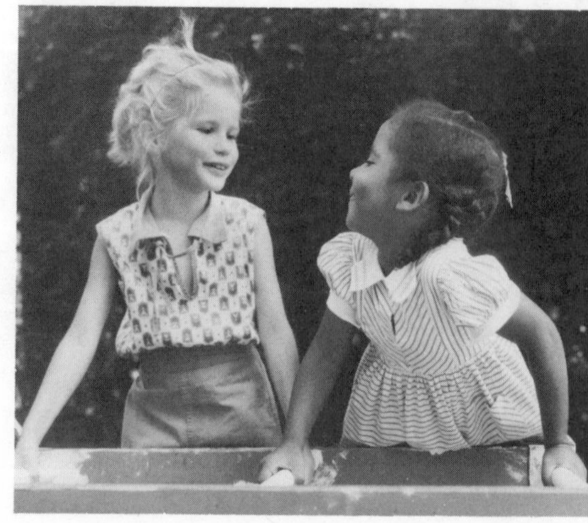

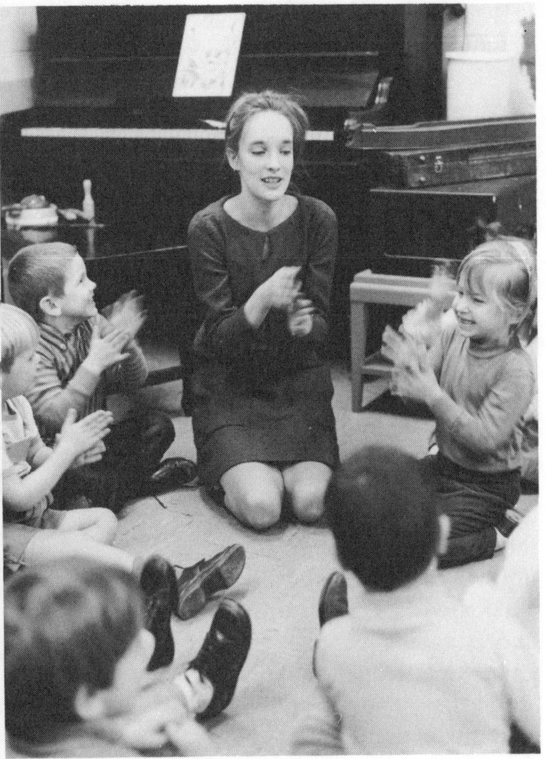

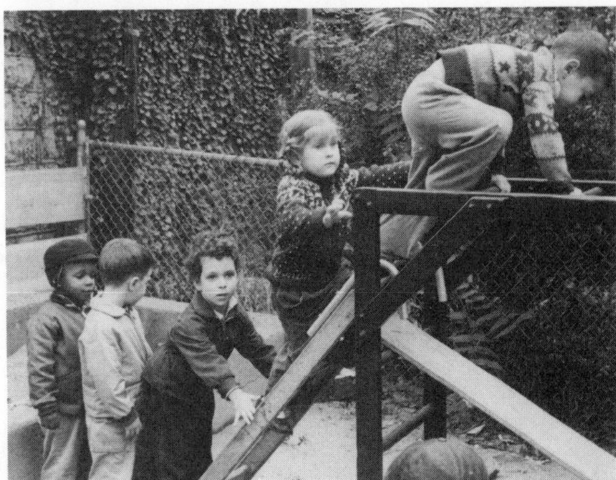

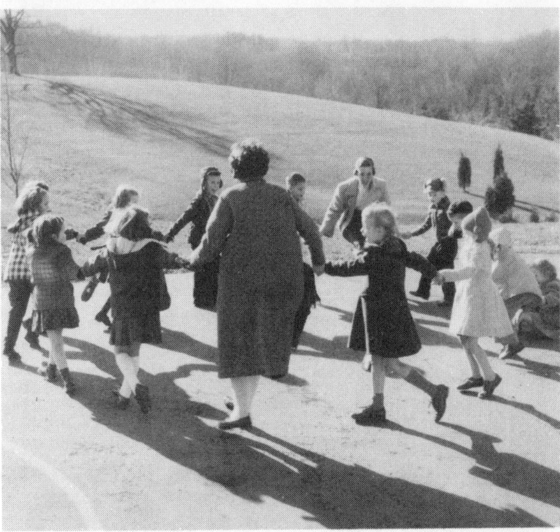

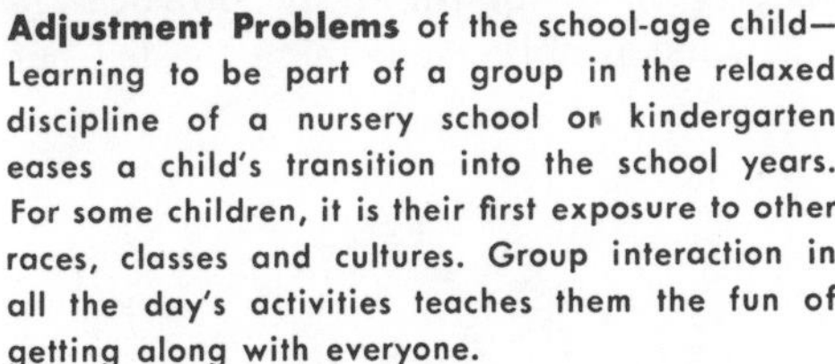

**Adjustment Problems** of the school-age child—Learning to be part of a group in the relaxed discipline of a nursery school or kindergarten eases a child's transition into the school years. For some children, it is their first exposure to other races, classes and cultures. Group interaction in all the day's activities teaches them the fun of getting along with everyone.

school and any difficulties associated with leaving home for the first time are smoothed out, parents tend to relax. For the first time in five or six years, the mother has several uninterrupted hours for herself, to spend at home or to use in her job or profession. The early school years may indeed be a relatively calm interlude between the nursery and adolescence, but even the normal healthy child has adjustments to make as he moves from home to school and from parental dependence to partial independence.

The first adjustment results from leaving home, for the first time, for an extended period. Usually, the first move is

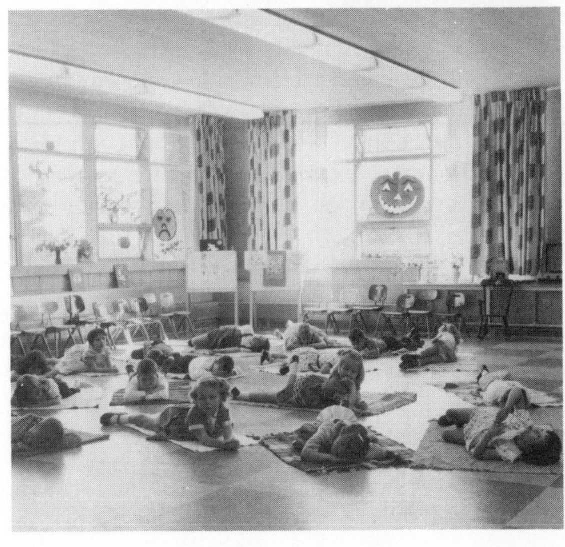

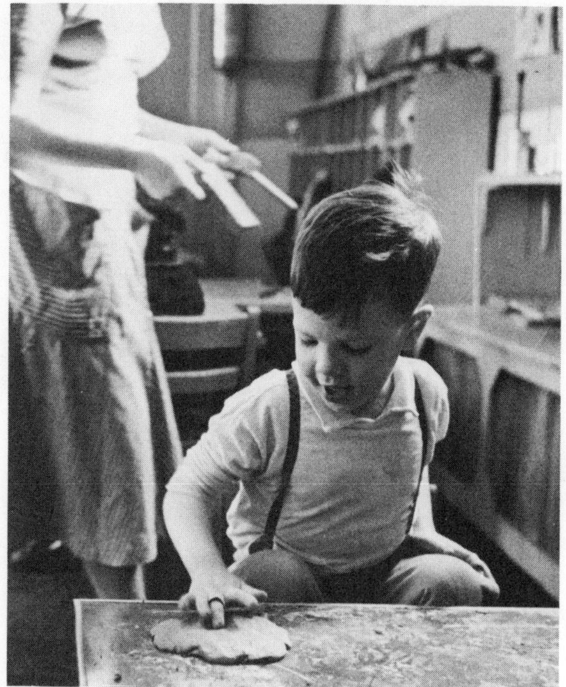

**Adjustment Problems** of the school-age child—Group play is valuable in a child's development. But periods of working independently, as above with modeling dough, are a welcome balance.

to nursery school or to kindergarten. The trend today is to begin education even earlier, and some parents arrange to have their children enrolled in a neighborhood "play school" for two or three hours a day. In any of these preschool settings, children are offered an easy transition from spending the entire day at home to being at school for as long as six hours. For many young children, whether they first leave home as early as age four or not until they enter first grade, health problems are directly related to the adjustment they must make. The child entering any new school setting must face a temporary separation from his mother, learn to get along with other children, and begin to learn in a formal way, contrasted with the informal and intuitive learning he had in his home.

A family doctor, pediatrician, or clinic physician or counselor can gauge the child's ability to make the adjustment to separation. In some schools, a counselor may be available to answer parents' questions and to refer the child, if necessary, to a doctor or psychologist for assistance. Although a group of youngsters on their way to school appear to be carefree, each of them comes from a different background and family circumstances, and some need help in adjusting.

Some children experience physical pain or other symptoms when it is time to enter school. They may have abdominal pain and feel nauseated. Some vomit when they leave the house or arrive at school. Some suffer nightmares or suddenly wet the bed for the first time in three or four years. These physical reactions to the anxiety of separation may be eliminated in a short time by gentle and understanding parents, or they may require professional attention.

Teachers know that six-year-olds have a short concentration span. Normally, they begin to squirm at any provocation —a sudden noise, something the teacher

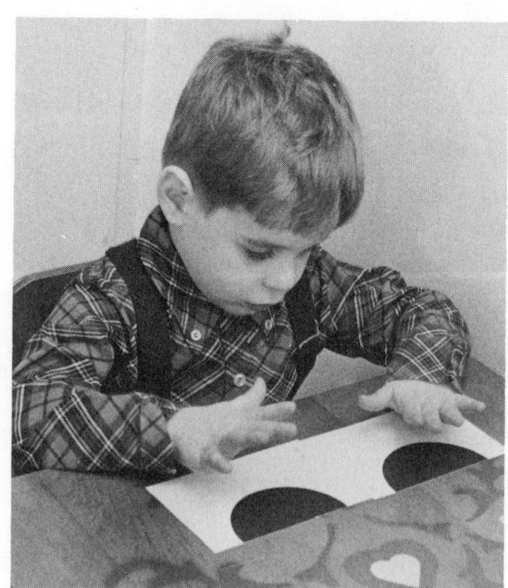

**Adjustment Problems** of the school-age child—A challenging task that is within a child's capabilities helps to maintain discipline in play school. An added reward will be the youngster's pride when he joins the two halves to shape a ball.

says, a whispered joke from one of the other children, or a dropped book. They giggle and talk out of turn. In more and more schools, classrooms are becoming less formal, to accommodate the natural energy, curiosity, and short attention span of young children. However, some children go beyond the normal stage of squirming and become so restless that they disturb the entire class and are themselves unable to concentrate on what the teacher is saying. A child who develops a *tic* (involuntary twitching movement) should be seen by a doctor. Some children outgrow tics, but others continue to display them into adolescence and adulthood. A much more serious condition is *chorea,* a nervous disease marked by involuntary jerking movements. In some types of chorea, speech disorders and muscular weakness also develop.

While almost all children are curious and eager when they enter school, too many soon become uninterested and complain of being tired or bored. Parents may examine the school situation carefully to determine the causes of slow learning. Some children do poorly in school because of pre-existing health problems that have been neglected or improperly treated. A problem of vision or hearing may be undetected until a child is in school and begins to have trouble learning to read. Special appraisal and treatment, tutoring, or other types of assistance may be necessary. Difficulties in the home may appear as difficulties in adjusting to school. Since reading is the first and most basic skill the child must acquire, difficulty or failure in this area demands immediate attention. A child's feeling of insecurity or inadequacy may underlie his reading difficulty. The earlier such an emotional problem is recognized and treated, the more optimistic is the outlook for the child's future.

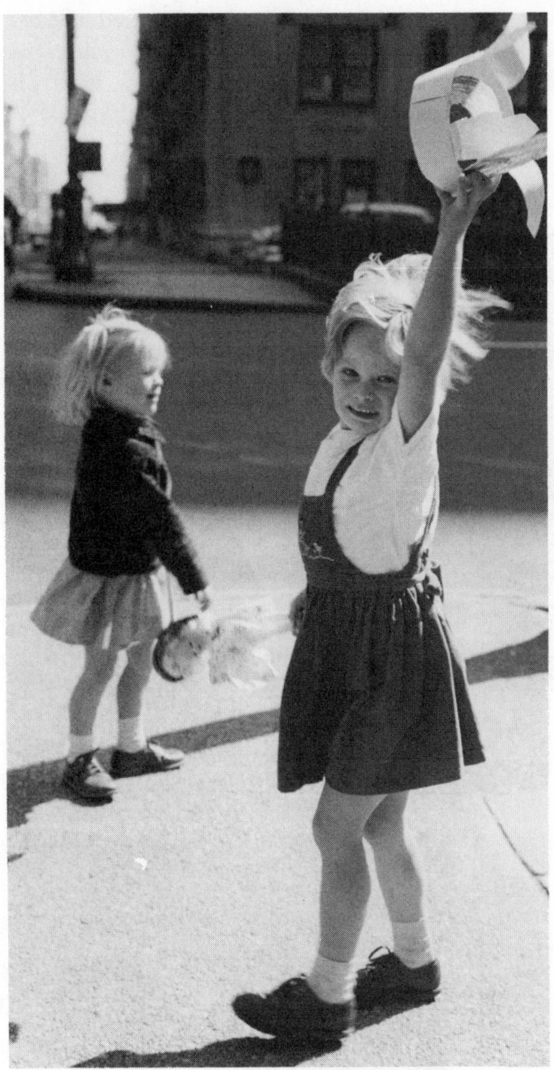

**Adjustment Problems** of the school-age child—On her way home from school, a child proudly displays the results of the day's work. This sense of achievement is important in helping children to develop positive attitudes about going to school in general and learning in particular. Tangible proof of progress compensates for the loss of the freedom of preschool days.

Adjustment problems of the school-age child require the utmost cooperation between parents and the skilled specialist who is called in to help the child. If a doctor's examination determines that physical problems are not causing difficulty in adjustment, the parents owe it to their child to be completely open and honest with the doctor so that the emotional difficulties can be identified and the child helped. The early school years can be rewarding for the child and his parents if the early adjustment problems are faced honestly and the child is helped to move toward independence, to work and play with his peers, and to learn up to his intellectual potential. *See also* ADOLESCENCE; ALEXIA; HYPERKINESIS; INTELLIGENCE.

▶ Sex and Sex Education, *Sex Education of Children,* 2643.

◆ The Child in the Family, 1781. First Steps to Childhood, 1789.

## THE CHILD IN SOCIETY

**Small children live in a tight, restricted world, their vision bound by simple stereotypes. But their needs are extremely complex and the degree to which they are met affects their entire future development.**

AS SOON AS BABIES BEGIN to be able to tell the difference between their own bodies and the world around them, they start to develop a sense of identity. As they grow out of babyhood, they extend their relationships. At first there is simply the mother and the child. Then the relationship is father, mother and child. Later brothers and sisters are included, and later still strangers and others with whom the child comes into contact.

The only adjustment these little girls had to make on meeting at play school was to learn each other's names. They are too young to let their racial difference matter or even to be aware of it.

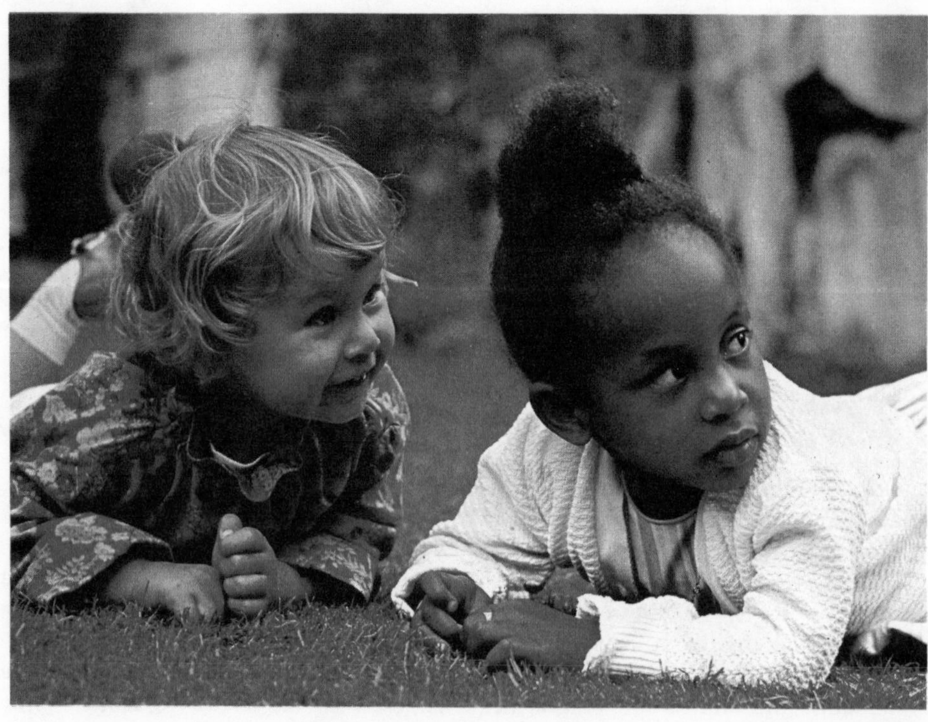

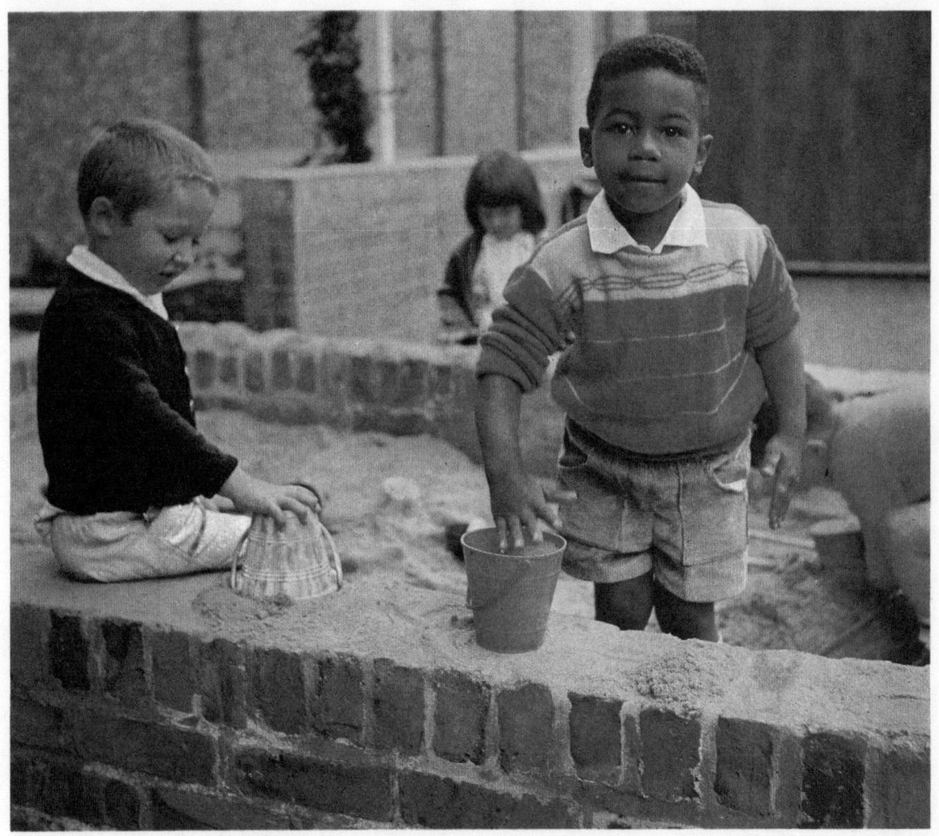

The playground is another area where children learn early the give and take of functioning in society. Some encounters are stormy, but most are as relaxed and friendly as the one above.

Children who live a very protected and sheltered existence or whose parents are socially isolated may meet few other people, or those they meet may all be of one type. But whether they actually meet them or not, as they grow they get impressions of people around them, put them into categories and get an idea of the larger world.

### THROUGH A CHILD'S EYES

Children develop these ideas not only on the basis of personal experience but also on the way in which parents, other children, teachers, and other adults think about and act towards people. By about seven, children often have a rudimentary idea of class, nation and race and are beginning to think in terms of accepted adult *stereotypes* about people. That is they can classify individuals according to very simple and often superficial ideas relating to the color of their skin, their social habits, their speech and dress. These stereotypes are rigid caricatures of what people are really like. The more socially insecure people are, the more they tend to think in these terms, because they give an illusion of safety in human relationships. Children's stories and comics, films, cartoons and jokes can reinforce these attitudes.

In this way, children may grow up in a tight little world of their own, limited by the walls of home and school and the geographical horizons which restrict their ex-

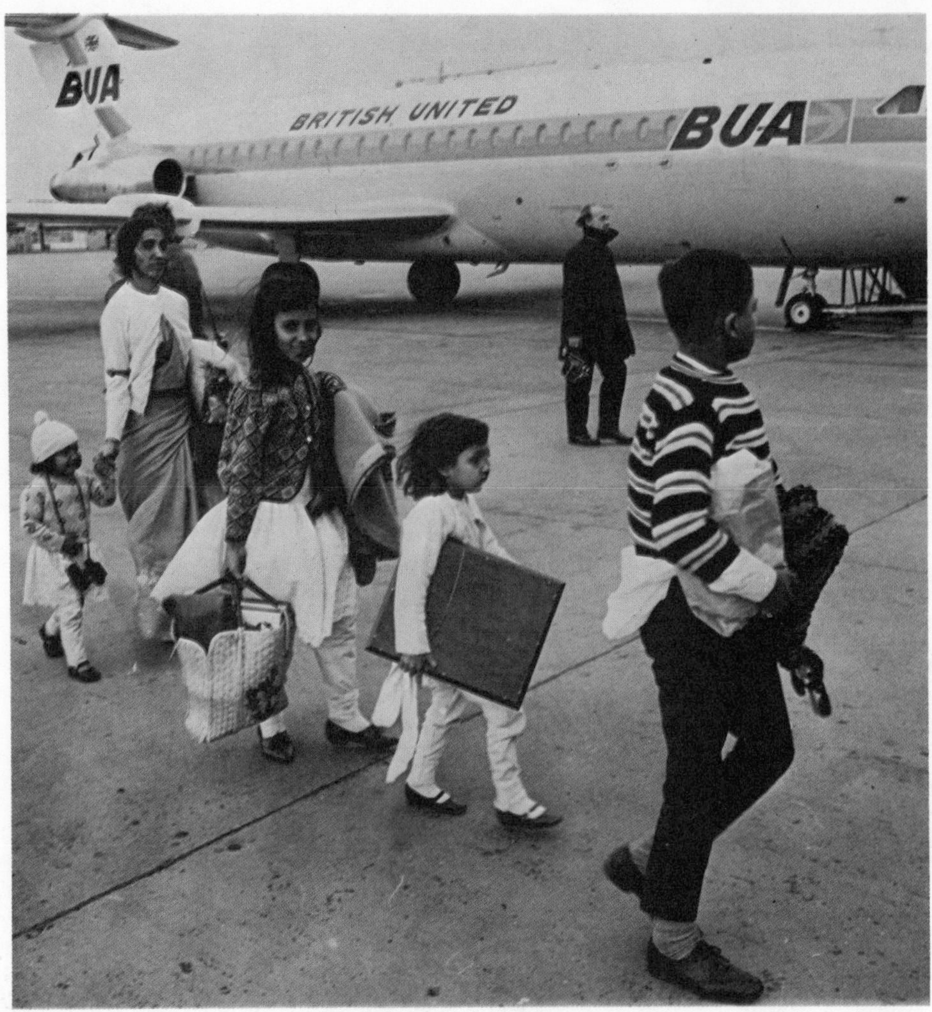


An Asian migrant family arrives in England full of hope for the future. Family members face major adjustments to alien customs and food and a sophisticated environment. The school-age children must further contend with studying in a new language, with children who may not accept them.

ploration, and by ideas and stereotypes which classify other people in the world around them. These factors also limit their opportunities for social contact. Stereotypes are not simply passive pictures, but are frequently signals for action and for certain kinds of social behavior; they usually trigger off reactions of contact with or rejection of the people concerned.

If children are asked whom they play with in the school playground, there will be some children who choose a large group, some who are chosen by more than one other child, combinations of these, and children who are quite alone, whom nobody chooses to play with—social outcasts. The choice of friends may depend almost entirely upon their personal qualities, but after about the age of seven children tend to choose friends who fit into certain classified categories in their own minds, and to exclude those who seem socially inferior or different.

Children of minority groups often grow up in situations of interracial stress and resulting insecurity and have problems over and above those which children face normally in growing up. Sometimes they are forced to confront open hostility, threats and even violence; sometimes it is rather a question of isolation through social distance. For those from foreign countries, to this are added language difficulties and family difficulties in adjusting to an alien culture.

Although children easily adopt the customs of their new country, this is harder for adults, and a gulf may be created between the first and second generation of an immigrant family. Members of what many sociologists call the *host society* tend to lump all immigrants together, unable or unwilling to understand the differences between them and to realize that they can come from widely varied cultural backgrounds. Some areas of the country are providing bilingual schooling to help ease the transition of immigrant children into American life. However, this must be combined with a study of English since that is the language in which most will be expected to function in their working lives in the United States.

## POVERTY'S CHILDREN

Since immigrants tend to be absorbed into an alien society at the lowest economic levels, many of their children are brought up in poverty—as are those of other minorities, who as a group were hit hardest by the American recession and inflation of the 1970s. They live in poor housing where there is overcrowding, inadequate sanitary facilities, cockroach and rat infestation and little or no privacy. Such situations are bound to have effects in the future. Childhood suffering is not something on which a grown person simply closes a door; experiences in childhood form an integral part of the adult's personality.

A particularly deprived minority are the children of migratory farm workers who harvest so much of the nation's food. The youngsters themselves usually work in the fields from an early age in order to boost the family's meager income. As they follow the seasonal harvesting from southern to northern areas, or from eastern to western farmlands, there is precious little time to get much schooling to prepare them for a more rewarding way of earning a living. Thus the dreary pattern repeats itself all too often and generation after generation is trapped in substandard housing and a threadbare way of life. Even the enormous social service programs of the federal government do not seem to touch their lives enough to break the circle of poverty.

## ILLEGITIMACY AND INTEGRATION

But a child does not have to look different, speak the wrong language, or live poorly to feel different from others. Adopted children who have not been given all the facts about their adoption may suffer great unhappiness and feelings of not belonging. Those who have been told the truth may be tormented by feelings of having been rejected by their real parents, and they too wonder where they belong. Illegitimate children not put up for adoption may become equally isolated.

Illegitimate births have soared in the past two decades, and the number of unwed mothers choosing to keep and raise their babies themselves has greatly increased. With the new freedom of the so-called sex revolution, for some there is no longer the stigma formerly attached to bearing a child out of wedlock and they feel they have nothing to hide.

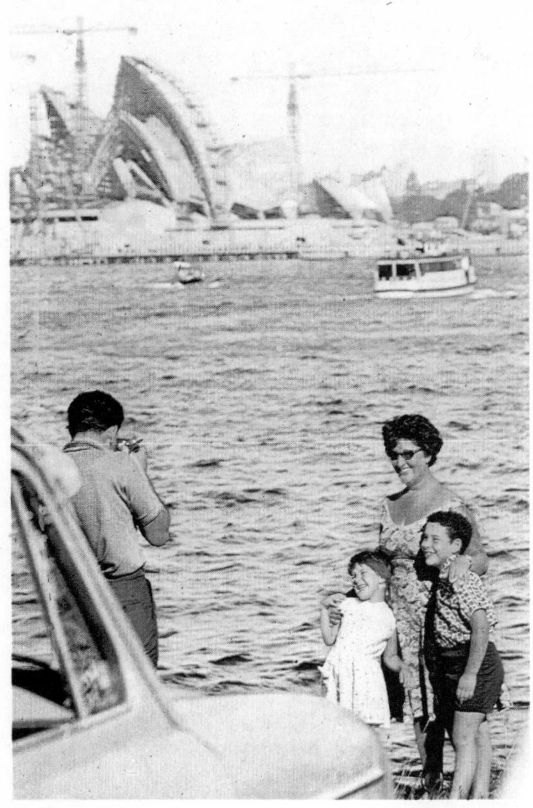

The children of this English family newly migrated to Australia have a major point in their favor as they go on with their lives. There is no language barrier to be overcome in their new country!

Unfortunately, many of these unwed mothers are too young and unskilled to support themselves and a child and both end up on welfare. So the child grows up fatherless *and* poor, forced to battle as it grows older for the respect often denied by children born within a marriage. And while to a lonely, perhaps neglected, 15-year-old girl a baby of her own may seem a special gift to fill her life, having the responsibility for a lively ten-year-old when she herself is only 25, or for a 15-year-old adolescent when she is just 30, may not be much fun at all—producing still more stress for the child.

Another addition to the stress of growing up has been the massive effort to integrate American schools. With black and white children being bussed in and out of urban and suburban areas—sometimes accompanied by heated resistance—new demands are made on their adaptability under pressure. The mixing of races is in many instances also a mixing of cultures and standards—with the inevitable conflicts produced by such meetings. Yet this same exposure is invaluable as a bridge to understanding between groups, the lack of which is most often the true cause of racism.

## CHILDREN WHO ARE NOT WELL

Physically and mentally handicapped children also face special problems as they grow up. Sometimes these are insuperable. They start off with an additional disadvantage, because mothers who bear such children often feel ashamed, even to the point of trying to hide the child and not letting friends and relatives know. Others feel a deep sense of guilt, and blame themselves for producing a deformed baby. This feeling of guilt may interfere with a mother's natural relationship with the child, so that she is anxious, devotes too much of her mental energies to its care, may be over-protective and devote so much time and attention to the child that she neglects her other children and her husband. This situation is understandable, since these children do need a great deal of care and attention if they are to develop their potentialities. But the feelings of a mother for her child may affect the ultimate success of any treatment, and they have been estimated as the most important single factor in that treatment.

As medical care improves, more and more children survive who at one time would have died during or shortly after birth, and new problems in rearing severely handicapped children are arising. These are not just medical problems but social problems, concerning everyone and attitudes to those in the community who have less than the normal chances of achievement.

Many children suffer because they are in some way different from others around them. A child who has eczema or pimples or who is especially fat may have a hard time facing social relationships. Obesity in children is becoming increasingly common, especially in the United States and Britain. In these countries, malnutrition (of a very different kind from that found in underdeveloped countries) is linked with modern habits of living. Children may be weaned straight on to ice cream, soft drinks, chocolate cookies and other carbohydrate foods, resulting not only in obesity but also in a high incidence of tooth decay.

This problem does not start with hungry school-age children. It has its beginnings in babyhood, and it has been shown by recent research that fat babies are likely to grow into fat children, and fat children into fat adults. A common cause is overfeeding of babies with patent baby cereals, by proud mothers competing with others to show how their offspring gain weight.

A deprived child is not necessarily a member of a racial minority, a child who lives in a slum, or a child who is motherless or handicapped in an obvious way. Many children of preschool age, and especially those from poor families, are deprived of opportunities for development through play, the company of other children and adults, and adequate space for uninhibited movement. The parents of such children may have adequate finances, but if they live in an area of high-rise apartments, all

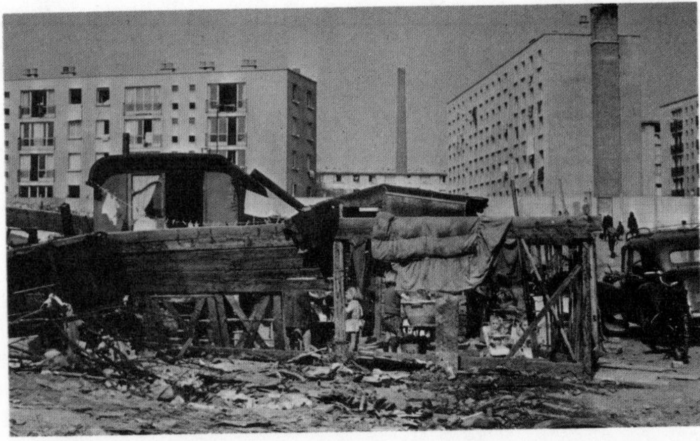

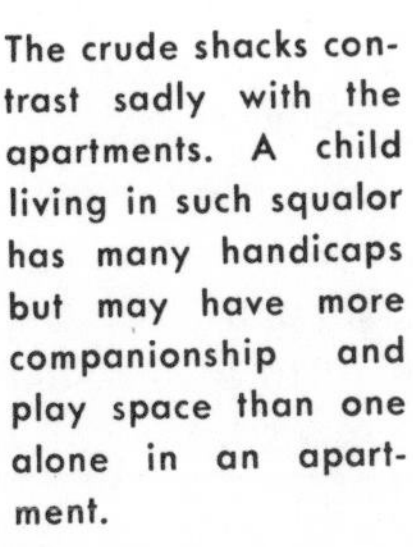

The crude shacks contrast sadly with the apartments. A child living in such squalor has many handicaps but may have more companionship and play space than one alone in an apartment.

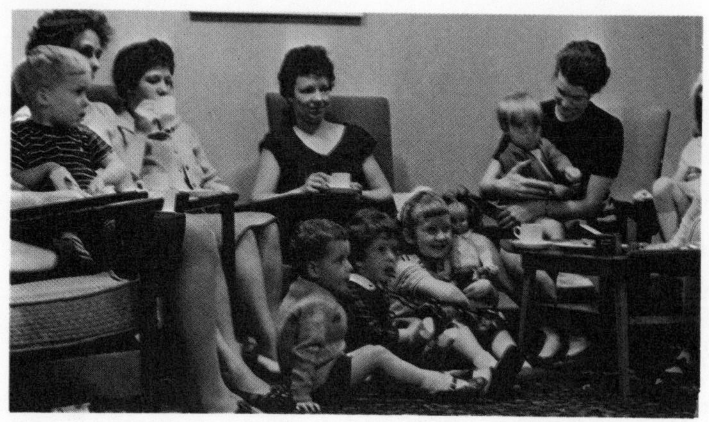

These children are making excellent progress after surgery. Loving care from mothers and substitute mothers helped overcome the trauma of hospitalization to promote faster recovery.

these conditions may be present and the child is no less deprived than one in a slum—who may, indeed, be surrounded by other children and the raw materials of play. The slum child could be far better off than the lonely child in an apartment.

### THE LONELY UNDER-FIVES

Nursery schools and the playgroup movement aim at enriching the lives of preschool children, offering a good environment for experiment, for making messes without anybody caring, and for learning about the world and other people.

A great many children grow up with no physical, mental or social handicaps, but nevertheless need special care. They may be children who have suffered some form of *maternal deprivation* between the ages of about six months and three years. This deprivation can happen through no fault of the mother; she may have had to enter a hospital for a long time, or have been unmarried and unable to keep the child permanently with her. Some children react violently to maternal absence by starting to wet the bed again, refusing to eat, or flying into tantrums. But these children can at least make their presence felt and make it clear that they do not like to be left. The children who suffer most are those who are unable to express themselves in this way and who quietly withdraw from human relationships. The mothers, too, suffer when they are cut off from contact with their children.

It has been found that a large proportion of juvenile delinquents had been separated from their mothers for six months or longer at some time between the ages of one and five. Another study revealed that a high proportion of patients receiving psychiatric care had suffered in early childhood from maternal deprivation through desertion, death or illness.

Researches in animal psychology may be important here. It has been shown that newly hatched chickens pass through a special period of development when they learn to follow their mother or any other individual—even a human being—who is present. Much the same happens to puppies aged between three and 13 weeks, after which age the capacity to form an attachment is much reduced. It looks as if there is a fairly short and highly critical period, similar to this "following response" demonstrated in birds and animals (which is called *imprinting*), when a child can form firm social attachments and close relationships with individuals. If that period is missed, the child may never again be able to enter satisfactorily into these sorts of relationships.

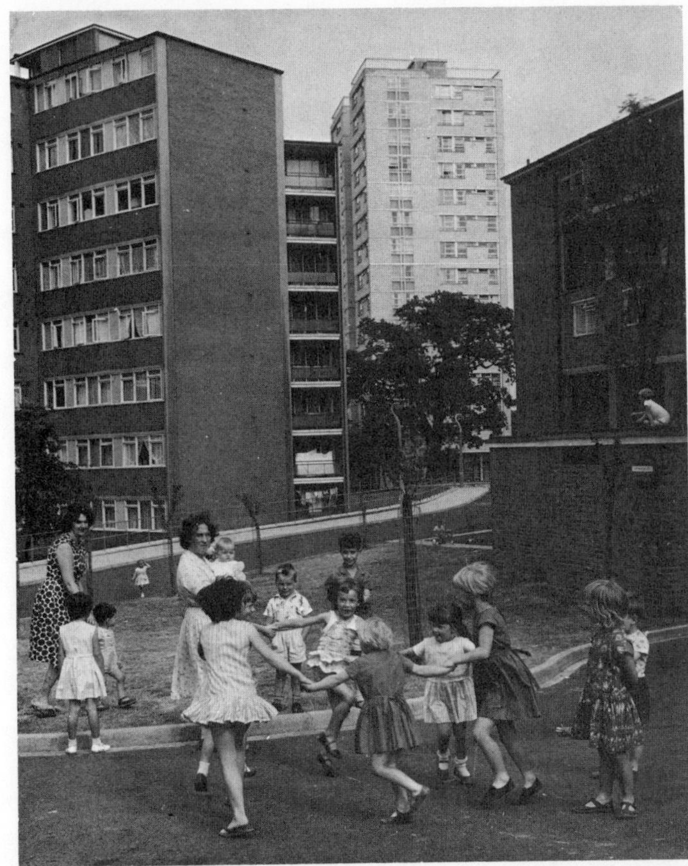

Outdoor play for small children can be a problem in high-rise apartment complexes. In some, mothers take turns supervising groups so that the children can have play time with friends.

These considerations are not meant to suggest that a mother can never leave her child. Rather, they suggest society should be organized in such a way that mothering tasks can be shared between mothers and fathers and between women who live in the same community, so that a small child need never be left completely alone for any length of time.

### EFFECTS OF HOSPITALIZATION

One of the ways in which a child often suffers from almost complete maternal deprivation is by being sent to a hospital. Just when the child is in pain and distress and most wants a mother's love and support, it may be cut off. The child is in a large building, surrounded by nurses and doctors who prod and examine and perform perhaps painful treatments. Reaction and adjustment to the strangeness of a hospital environment and the separation from mother and other family members will depend largely on a child's age and stage of development, the reason for the hospitalization, the hospital itself, and the preparation given the child by the parents and hospital staff.

The reason for the hospitalization and what will be done about it should be described in terms that will not frighten or confuse children. They also need reassurance that medicines, injections and other treatments are to make a child better so that he or she can go home as soon as possible. An explanation of hospital routine and equipment, that there will be other children there, and that there will be nurses around all the time to take care of them will help dispel a child's fear of the unknown.

In instances of emergency hospitalization, an extra effort must be made by parents to help the child and hospital staff adjust to each other. Staying with the child as much as possible—with parents perhaps taking turns so that one of them is there most of the time—is an invaluable aid in getting the child over the early stages of recovery.

Once hospitalization takes place, parents must then come to terms with a child in pain or discomfort, or the frustration and boredom a child feels when confined to bed or perhaps encumbered with an arm, leg or body cast. An intelligent mixture of sympathy, patience and common sense will help maintain the child's morale and promote a better emotional recovery from the trauma of illness and hospitalization.

**ADNEXA,** the adjoining or accessory parts of an organ. For example, *adnexa oculi* are the tear ducts and eyelids, and the *adnexa uteri* are the ovaries and Fallopian tubes.

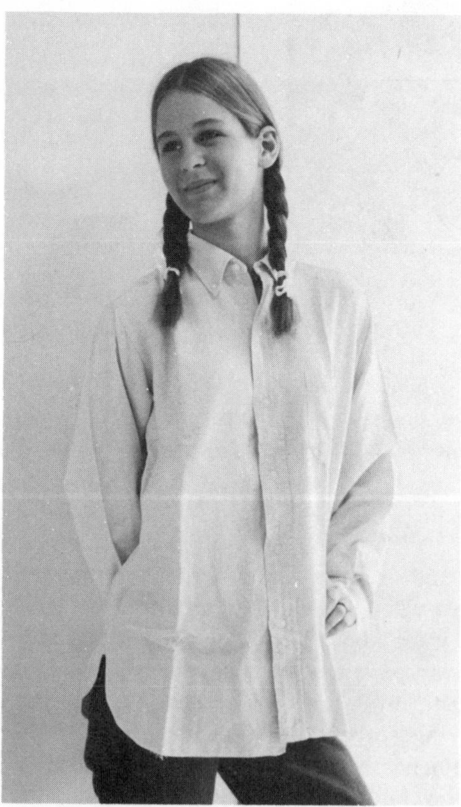

**Adolescence**—Because they are so sensitive about how they look, adolescents are quick to adopt hair and clothing fads. To look like everyone else gives them a needed sense of belonging.

**ADOLESCENCE,** the period of eight to ten years from *puberty* to full physical growth and maturity. The duration of adolescence differs; it usually begins at approximately 11 or 12 years in girls and at about 13 or 14 in boys. Adolescence does not end only when physical growth stops; the emotional turbulences associated with the period must subside and the individual be psychologically equipped to assume the responsibilities of adult life. For some persons, adolescence is over by age 18. For others, it lingers on into the 20's.

Except for the first year of life, at no other time does a boy or girl grow and change so much and in so many ways as during adolescence. Glandular activity increases, bringing about growth and sexual maturity. The long bones grow rapidly and the muscles increase in size and strength. The thyroid gland enlarges, sometimes so much (especially in a slender individual) that it looks like a *goiter*. The primary sex organs mature and secondary sexual characteristics appear. Voices—most noticeably those of boys—change to their adult sound. The skin is affected by the overproduction of the oil glands, and *acne* often becomes an annoying problem. Adolescent boys and girls virtually rebuild their childhood bodies into new ones, to which they must become gradually accustomed.

Since so much happens so fast, the boy or girl is not prepared. Young teen-

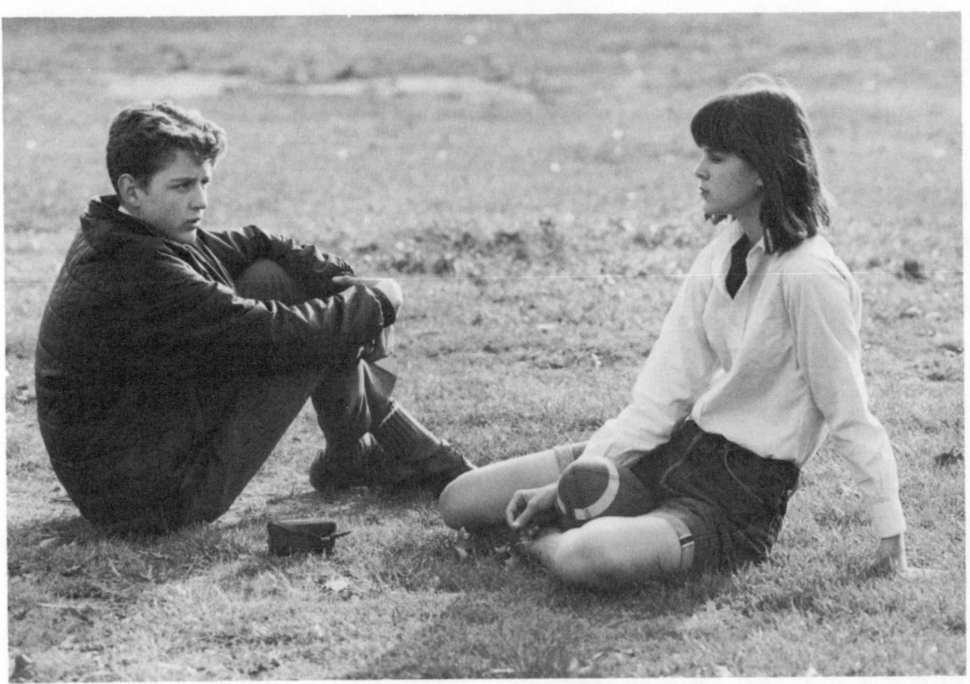

**Adolescence**—Young teenagers often feel better able to share problems and ideas with each other than with adults. But it is important to keep lines of communication open with parents as well. Mutual tolerance and patience help soothe the inevitable frictions between generations.

agers are worried and preoccupied about the physical changes they undergo. They incessantly compare themselves to other boys and girls their own age, and wonder if everything about them is "right." Adolescents are extremely sensitive about how they look. They should never be ridiculed or embarrassed about their appearance, habits, feelings, or choice of clothing. Adolescents not only develop at different rates, but growth in each rarely proceeds in a coordinated way. A boy may grow several inches in a year without putting on a proportionate amount of weight, so that he appears temporarily gawky and awkward. A girl's sex organs may develop quickly and her menstrual periods begin, but she may be worried because her breasts are not as full as she thinks they should be. Youngsters may go through a stage of being underweight, then overweight, before their growth tapers off and a combination of correct diet and exercise enables their bodies to take on an attractive mature appearance.

Matters that most concern adolescents are sex, the loosening of family ties, the growth of independence, and gaining recognition and acceptance by their peers. In these, as in questions of physical health, the role of adults—and especially of parents—is not to shield adolescents from difficult experiences, but to proffer assistance when it is needed, always understanding that this is a troublesome time for boys and girls. Adolescence is a difficult time for parents too, for they must be able to reassure their children of their love and protection while acknowledging that these same children are growing up and becoming independent self-sufficient adults.

Sex is one of the most baffling problems for teenagers. They are becoming physiologically mature, their sex drive is reaching its lifetime peak, and they are

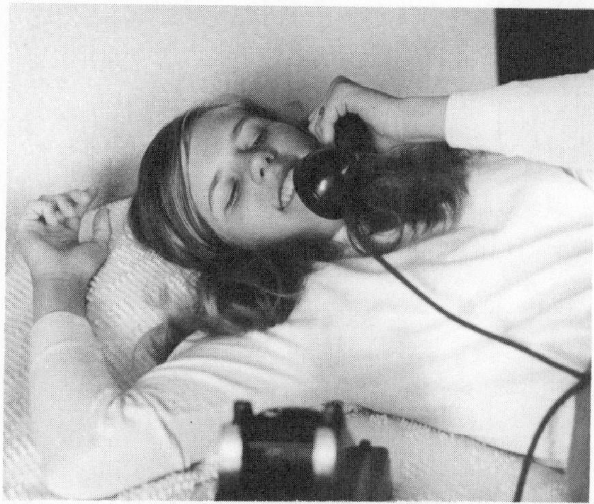

**Adolescence**—Perhaps because it lets them say things they would be too shy to say in person, teenagers love talking on the telephone. But they must learn to share it with other family members.

acutely aware of the differences between what they may have heard at home and school concerning acceptable social behavior, and what they find actually takes place around them. The contemporary libertarian attitude about sex and the growing toleration of premarital sexual intercourse are not necessarily immediately acceptable to every adolescent. A new freedom can be a source of anxiety. Many teenagers who brag about their sexual exploits are secretly confused about their sexual development, uncertain of their appeal to the opposite sex, and muddled about their feelings and attitudes toward sexuality. Hero worship, romantic attachments, a "crush" on someone of the same sex—sometimes involving a peer and sometimes a respected adult—are normal during adolescence. Strong boy-boy and girl-girl attachments are a healthy and temporary phase. Parents should not become anxious and label these as homosexual, nor should they make their children anxious about them. Only if this phase becomes unusually intense and lasts a long time need parents become concerned. They should discuss the matter with their doctor or clergyman privately to try to gauge the legitimacy of their concern, rather than immediately make their child feel that something is wrong with him or her.

The changing relationships to their parents are important to adolescents. They rely less on their mothers and fathers and more on their friends, who cling together for mutual protection and assurance. Hesitant about standing alone and defiant about being considered children, adolescents go through trying times as they work their way through the years of growing up. Adolescents need to achieve independence, although the rebellious process of doing so may be unpleasant for everyone concerned. Parents can help their teenage boys and girls far more by encouraging them in their maturity than by taking from them the confidence they need if they are to succeed. The most rebellious boys and girls—those who are the most argumentative, sullen, or unpleasant—may be those who suffer the most insecurity about leaving the protection of childhood. Patience and tolerance under trying circumstances are not easy for parents to achieve, but these qualities are vital in reassuring the adolescent that he is accepted.

Some medical problems afflict both boys and girls during adolescence. If they are underweight, they may lack the energy to take part in activities they enjoy and may have lowered resistance to disease. *Tuberculosis* is a potential threat to underweight adolescents, who also may not be getting a healthful diet. Overweight boys and girls suffer because they often are ridiculed and cannot participate in teenage activities. They may eat even more because of frustration and anger, and the cycle becomes difficult to break. Diet is especially important during adolescence. Parents who detect a weight problem, evidence of being overtired, an unusual number of colds, or other deviations from their children's normal physical condition, should consult a doctor. The rapid growth and strenuous exercise typical of adolescence calls for a complete diet, rich in protein for muscular and tissue growth, minerals for sturdy skeletal development, and enough carbohydrates and fat for energy. A doctor may advise vitamin supplements, but neither children nor their parents should undertake a vitamin regimen without medical approval.

Skin problems are especially prevalent. *Acne* is the most common skin ailment of adolescence, but boils and other skin complaints often plague teenagers. Severe cases of acne should be referred to a dermatologist. Mild cases can be handled by scrupulously keeping the skin clean and being alert to foods that set off a flare-up of acne. Girls should avoid heavy cosmetics that clog the pores.

One of the infections most prevalent among adolescents is *infectious mononucleosis* (*glandular fever*). The exact cause is thought to be a viral microorganism. Typical symptoms are extreme fatigue, a low fever—about 100-101°F—mild headache, and sore throat. Sometimes, there is nausea and vomiting, plus a loss of appetite. Mononucleosis may last up to six weeks. During this time, lymph nodes in the head and armpit become enlarged and there may be upper abdominal pain. The most effective treatment is bed rest and a medically supervised diet. Antibiotics may be used.

*Special Problems of Adolescent Girls.* As the *ovaries* (female sex glands) mature, a girl's body changes markedly. Her hips become rounder, and her breasts develop. Girls who develop quickly may be uncertain or embarrassed and may develop a poor posture in an attempt to hide their appearance. Mothers can help their daughters by explaining how these bodily changes are a preparation for womanhood, and can also guide them in their choice of more grown-up clothes.

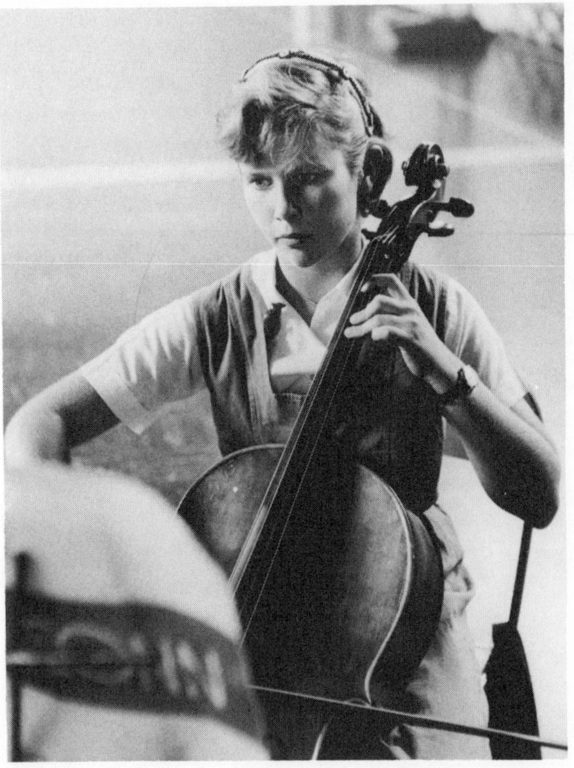

**Adolescence**—The satisfaction and prestige of playing an instrument in the school orchestra or band has made life bearable for many an adolescent—one reason musically inclined children should be encouraged to develop their talents.

*Menstruation* may precede, accompany, or follow other bodily changes. The onset of menstruation usually occurs between 12 and 14 years of age, but may start as early as 10 or be delayed as late as 16 or 17. In addition to needing help with the special emotional difficulties that may accompany the beginning of menstruation, a girl should see a doctor if her periods are painful and difficult. Adolescent menstruation is often irregular, but irregularity itself should not be a cause for concern. Menstruation normally occurs every 28 days and lasts from 3 to 7 days. The cycle can range from every 20 to every 35 or 40 days. Some adolescents menstruate only every two or three months, especially if they are under emotional stress. In most such cases, their doctor will tell them that there is no physical disorder.

A girl should be told about menstruation before it is likely to occur. Otherwise, her first period (*menarche*) can be frightening. In many societies, menstruation is considered a "curse," and even today, some parents in our society avoid discussing it, thereby letting their daughter think it is shameful. A girl should be encouraged to go about her normal home, school, and social activities unless her menstruation is especially painful. If she tires or chills easily, she should avoid swimming and the more strenuous sports during her period.

Mothers should instruct their daughters in the proper use of sanitary protection. Their doctor can help girls decide between internal and external devices and pads.

An adolescent girl may require an iron supplement in her diet if she has *anemia* associated with her menstrual period. Sufficient iron is contained in an adequate diet, but adolescent girls often follow a fad diet that may be deficient in iron and other substances required for good health.

**Adolescence**—The crucial teen years in rural areas benefit enormously from the agricultural programs of the 4-H Club. Two members proudly display steers they are raising as a 4-H project.

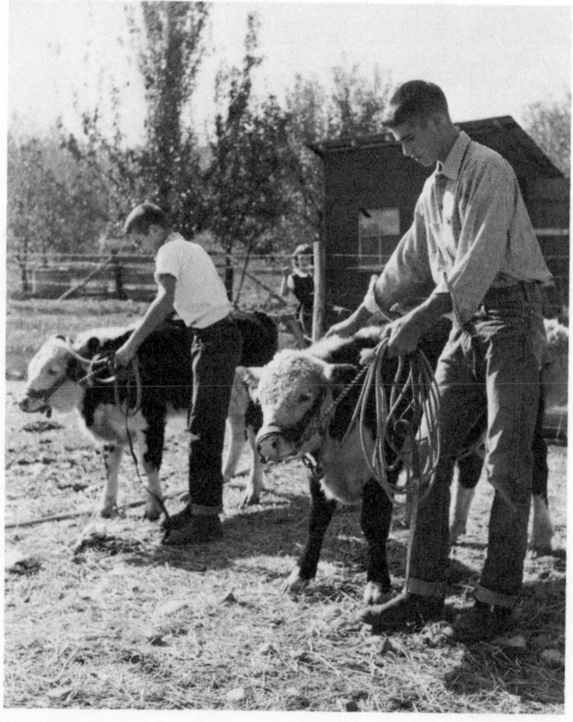

*Special Problems of Adolescent Boys.* Growth of the sex organ (*penis*) and the sex glands (*testes*) is one of the first signs of male adolescence. The testes produce a hormone (*testosterone*) that stimulates secondary sex characteristics, including the growth of hair under the arms, in the genital region, and on the face. When the testes are mature, they begin to produce sperm cells, and the boy is capable of ejaculation. Between the ages of 13 and 15, a boy may suddenly have an ejaculation or "wet dream" during sleep, accompanied by a sexual dream. Just as a girl should be told ahead of time by her mother about menstruation, so should a boy be told by his father to expect this *nocturnal emission*. He especially needs to be reassured that this is normal, healthy, and an important sign that he is becoming an adult. The sexual stimulations a young boy receives and the intensity of his response are individual. Parents need to know their son well to judge if his sexual development is within the wide range of normal, or whether either insufficient development or unusually vivid sexual fantasies and associated masturbation should be discussed with a doctor.

*Adolescents and the Doctor.* Even healthy adolescents should see a doctor annually, for a check on their physical and emotional growth and advice on maintaining their good health. Adolescents usually prefer to "graduate" from the pediatrician who has been seeing them since birth. They want to see their doctor in private and to have their confidences respected, just as doctors respect the information adult patients give them. Adolescent medicine has now developed into a recognized subspecialty. The physician may be a general practitioner or an internist, but he is prepared to recognize and treat the special disorders and problems of adolescents sympathetically.

Teenagers need to assume responsibility for their own health. If they can visit their own doctor, speak freely, and have their discussion held in confidence, they are more likely to respond positively to the advice the doctor gives them. Questions about a spot on the skin, a pain, sexual growth, questions that an adolescent wants very much to discuss but feels that he cannot do so freely with his parents, can be discussed openly in a doctor's office. An adolescent patient will generally understand that the conversation is in confidence, but that his parents must have enough information to follow through with any special treatment that the doctor prescribes. In this relationship—as in the adolescent's relationships with his parents and with his friends—the attitudes and feelings expressed and communicated are of utmost importance in helping the boy or girl live through these eight or ten years of remarkable growth in good health and with emotional security and resilience. *See also* PUBERTY.

▶ The Health of Women, *Puberty,* 1397; *Menstruation,* 1399. Psychiatry, *Therapy at Various Ages,* 2441. Sex and Sex Education, *Sex Education of Children,* 2643. The Importance of Skin, *Skin and Adolescence,* 2708.

◆ Reaching for Maturity, 1526.

## WHO IS THE ADOLESCENT?

**At adolescence, people start to explore and make a new world—new clothes, new music, new interest in the world's problems. Often, this stage in development leads to conflict within families.**

PRACTICALLY EVERYONE CONCERNED must adjust to some degree during that emotional and physical transition from childhood to adulthood called adolescence. The emerging adults—the teenagers—find life fairly exploding with new feelings, physical changes and growth, a developing sense of self, and a new freedom of movement. Their task is to adjust to all of these and at the same time come to terms with parents, teachers and friends on a new level.

A turbulent adolescence is considered by many to be inescapable in industrialized Western societies—both because of the relatively slow passage from childhood to adulthood that is permitted and the complexities of those societies. That adolescence is not a time of unrelieved anguish and frustration for everyone was established by a recent study of a group of middle-class boys aged 14–22. It showed three different types of development, with family lives a marked influence in each grouping.

One group progressed with calm self-assurance toward a meaningful and rewarding adult life. These boys had shown strength in earlier developmental stages and came from stable families that had not been subjected to major upsetting happenings—such as serious illness or death. Another group functioned well but the boys were subject to more conflicts in dealing with the problems of adolescent growth. These were more likely to come from families traumatized by serious disruptions such as death, illness or unusual separation.

The emotional growth pattern of the third group mirrored the popular concept of adolescence—much confusion and agitation, illustrated usually by difficult behavior at home and in school. Family lives of these boys had been weakened—such as by

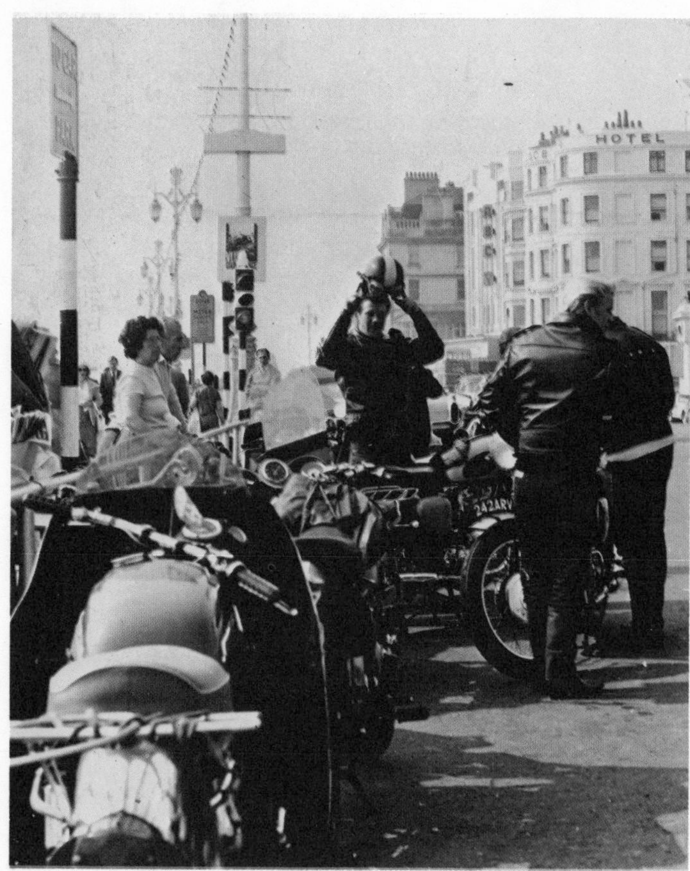


One youthful rebellion against society has been the motorcycle gangs that first erupted in the 1950's in the wake of rock 'n' roll. They roar through towns intent on speed, noise and sometimes violence, relishing the power of their disruptive behavior.

mental illness or obvious marital problems—and communication between parents and sons was inadequate or missing.

Where girls have been included in studies, results tend to suggest an adolescence more difficult than that of boys. Also, successful women more often than not will have had a rough adolescence, while girls with a fairly smooth adolescence have grown up to be somewhat depressed.

### TEENAGE TRAITS

Among the stronger psychological features of adolescence are a desire to conform with one's fellow teenagers in dress and behavior, a contrariness in dealing with parents and teachers, and a lack of confidence in themselves. All three seem to feed on one another and are aggravated by a general sense of anxiety. Unsure teenagers feel most able to contend with others of the same age and tend to resent those who have power over them. Hence, for their friends' approval and to demonstrate their freedom from childhood dependence, they usually indulge in some form of rebellion. This can range from staying out too late or playing hooky from school to far more serious acts such as the use of drugs or alcohol and robbery. How individual adolescents react depends largely on the sort of friends they have, the upbringing they have had and the neighborhood in which they live. For good or bad, adolescents have a great influence on each other and the common excuse is "everybody else is doing it."

One desirable result of wanting peer approval is the wish to excel in sport. The adolescent is likely to be near the peak of excellence in sport, and the desire to excel is in part related to a striving for approval among contemporaries.

THE DRUG PERIL

Earlier and heavier drinking and widespread drug use among today's adolescents is a devastating problem for more and more families. A recent study revealed that of 10,000 New York City public high school students questioned, 80 percent of 16-to-19-year-olds were drinking to some extent, and 12 percent could be classified as problem drinkers. On a larger scale, one estimate asserts that a serious drinking problem afflicts as many as 1.3 million 12-to-17-year-old Americans. The problem extends, of course, beyond the fact of drinking itself—teenagers represent 60 percent of those killed nationwide in accidents caused by drunken driving.

Adolescent drug use—barely heard of a generation ago—has grown alarmingly. For instance, from 1973 to 1975, marijuana use more than doubled among 14- and 15-year-olds (10 percent to 22 percent), and among the nation's high school seniors at least half had experimented with marijuana and six percent smoked it daily. One source of drugs for teenagers is the unscrupulous "pusher" who uses teenagers and even those not yet in their teens to sell drugs in areas around schools.

In addition to counseling, schools are trying to combat the destructive trend to drug abuse by having recovered addicts speak to the students. This enables them to hear first hand—and often from someone very close to their own age—the terrible physical and mental effects on young lives and the stupidity of drug abuse. Also, local social service agencies are sponsoring sessions where groups of teenagers and parents can meet and share their feelings and problems, guided by trained personnel.

A gaudily decorated young man personifies the relentlessly uninhibited behavior of some of the youth of the sixties. "Do your own thing" became the slogan and many young people forsook traditional values to live, work and dress in highly unconventional ways.

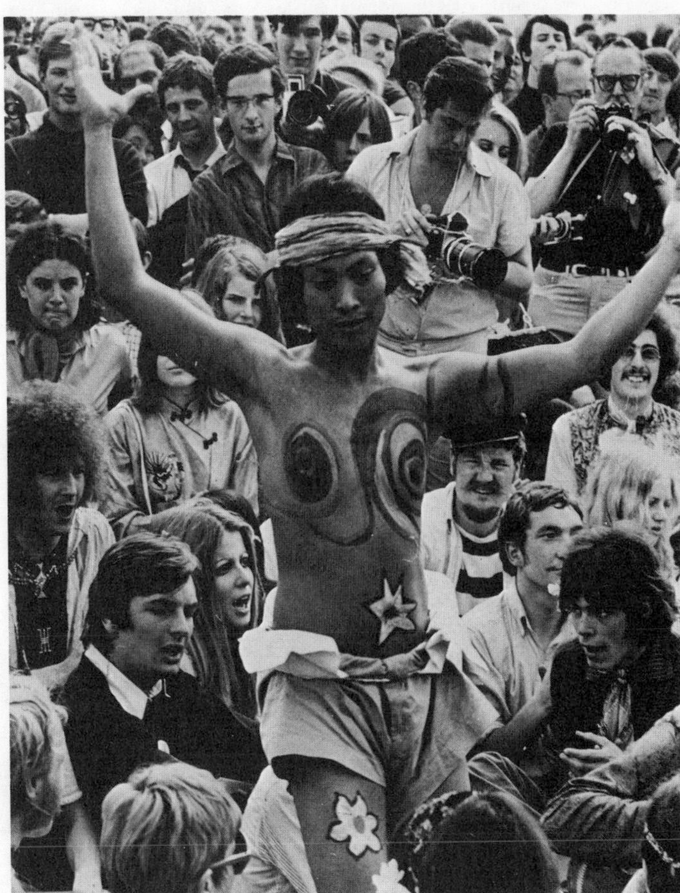

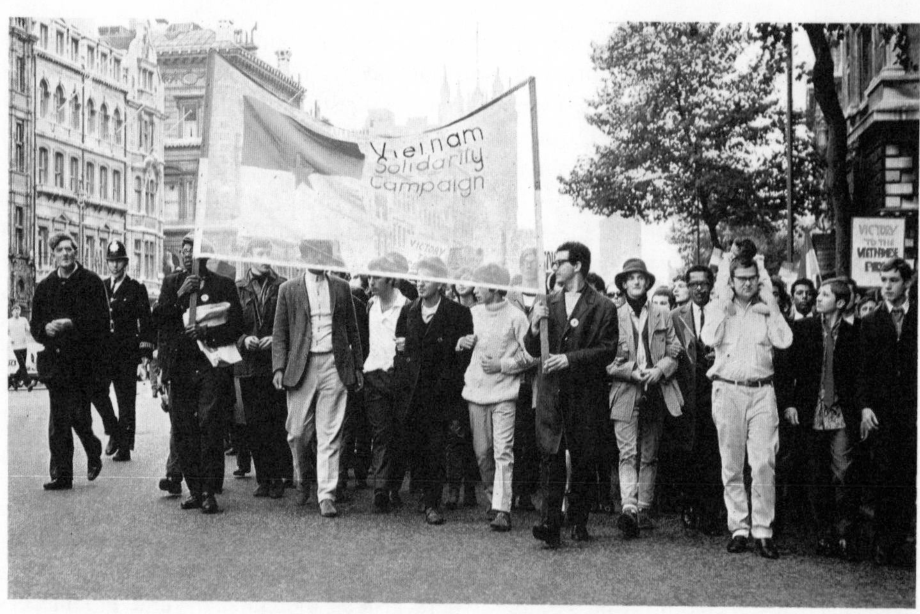


Two contrary aspects of adolescent behavior are an almost slavish adherence to fads and the sometimes strident assertions of independence. Participating in demonstrations, such as the march above in London to protest the Vietnam War, is one way youths feel they are publicly expressing their own opinions. Yet adolescents greatly influence each other and are quick to follow new trends in clothing and hairdos, however outlandish, such as the two below in the center.

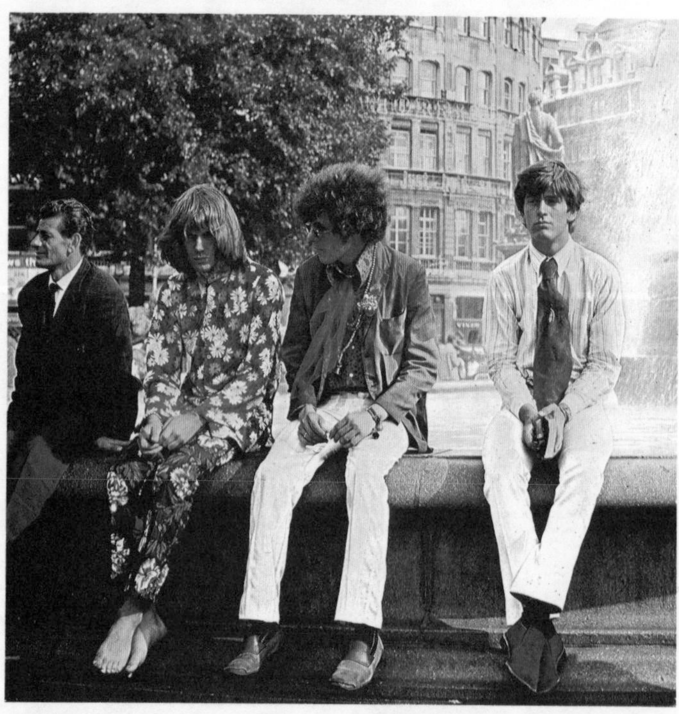

### ADOLESCENT SUICIDE

Then there are the teenagers who simply cannot make it at all. Among adolescents, suicide is the second most common cause of death—only accidents take more young lives. The suicide rate among Americans 13–19 years old almost doubled in the decade 1966–1976—from 1.7 to 3.1 per 100,000. In that same ten-year span, suicides among West German teenagers averaged about 500 a year. The frequent cause there seems to be the stress of demanding school examinations. Similarly, an intensely pressurized striving for university acceptance is blamed for the disproportionately high rate of suicide among young people in Japan. In the United States, the cause is often also tied to fears of failing in school or in college acceptance while under pressure from parents who want their children to do as well as or a lot better than they did. Other young people become severely depressed by feelings of inadequacy and rejection by their friends and schoolmates.

Suicide prevention centers have been organized in this country to contend with the general acceleration in that form of death. There are also "hot lines" and crisis lines in high schools, colleges and within communities.

### PUTTING SEX IN ITS PLACE

It is obvious and natural that adolescents should have a profound interest in sex, having undergone such marked changes in their sexual make-up. This usually develops in three phases. The first interest is in their own bodies and genital development, then there is a curiosity about bodies of those of the same sex, and finally the interest and energies turn to members of the opposite sex. This is, of course, one of the most potent developments of adolescence and one of the most difficult for parents and teenagers to handle.

During puberty, boys and girls tend to shun each other's company. However, with adolescence they acquire a new hobby—the opposite sex—and pursue it tirelessly. Relationships that result range from the frivolous, below, to genuine affection, with many variations in between.

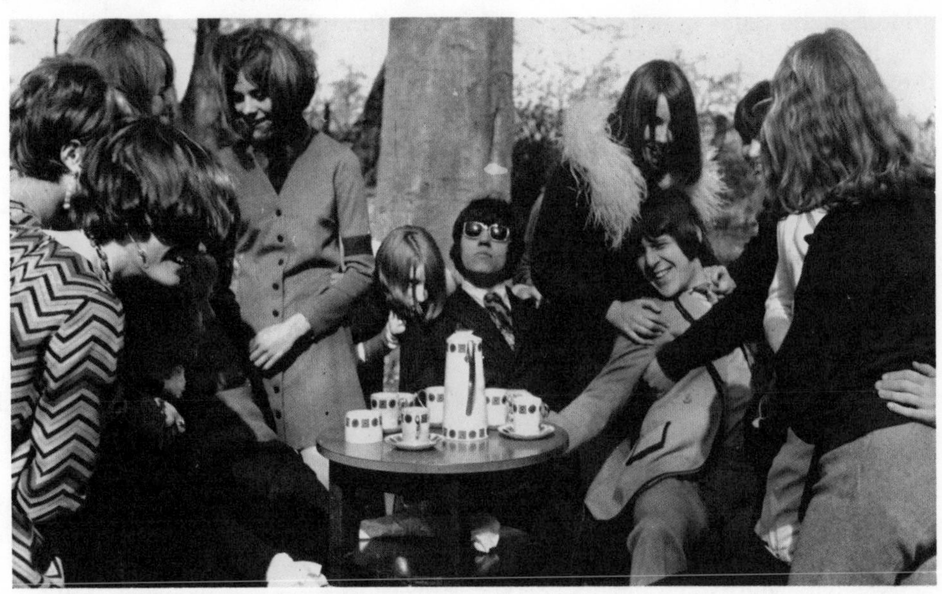

Today's permissive atmosphere has added further stress to the attractions, hopes, rivalries, successes and disappointments that have always characterized adolescent romance. Again, peer pressure and the everyone-is-doing-it argument can create enormous conflicts. Whether to engage in sexual activity or not, worry about possible venereal disease and pregnancy, and how to obtain contraceptives are added burdens for people still too inexperienced to make reasonable choices. At a time when unfortunately many parents seem to be adding their own permissiveness to that of society in general, adolescents are sorely in need of firm but understanding guidance.

Parents (or guardians) have the responsibility to give teenagers clear information about the changes taking place in their bodies, matters of health and hygiene, and above all to stress that they must learn to be responsible for their actions. It is their task to help the adolescents develop a mature and responsible code of behavior, sexual and otherwise. Parents also owe growing children a balanced, healthy home atmosphere in which to develop so that their advice is not lost in a maze of insecurities and antagonisms.

### ENERGY AND ENNUI

Restlessness, boredom and a disinclination to work are other common features of adolescents. Many are confused about which career to pursue, others may resist having to study when enjoying an active social life, and most tend to be easily bored by work, friends and family. Daydreaming is characteristic of the age. It is bound up with boredom, thoughts of happier days or more interesting pursuits and lack of discipline. All of this may lead to dropping out of school and the resulting loss of chances for a higher education. This can be a tragedy when the adolescent is of high intelligence and has prospects for an excellent future.

Though it is true that at puberty a boy or girl is beginning to desire some degree of privacy, and may become something of a lone wolf, the young adolescent is inclined to join groups of one kind or another—religious, political, or social. It is part of the desire to conform, but also part of the adolescents' intensity of feeling—about social issues, war and peace, sexual matters or so much that they feel is wrong in the world of adults. Some have the burning urge to reform the world and join groups of young people who think the same way.

Boys and girls at this age also have emotional ups and downs with rapid changes from laughter to withdrawal. Adolescents are particularly sensitive to comments from parents and others, and are easily offended, taking everything said as implying criticism. They are particularly likely to be infuriated by parental criticisms of their clothes, appearance, hair style, or, still more, of their friends. Failure of the parents to appreciate the sensitiveness of the adolescent is one of the major causes of friction at home.

### PARENT-CHILD FRICTION

Friction between teenagers and parents is very common. It certainly does not occur in all homes and it can certainly be avoided if parents are wise, tactful, tolerant and understanding in their dealings with their teenage sons and daughters.

Not unnaturally, many parents find it difficult to relax discipline, to balance overprotection with unjustifiable carelessness. If they go too far one way the adolescent rebels; if they go too far the other way he or she may get into trouble. For example, it is not easy for a teenage girl to accept the injunction that she cannot hitch-hike. She lacks the maturity and the necessary experience to know that the dangers are too

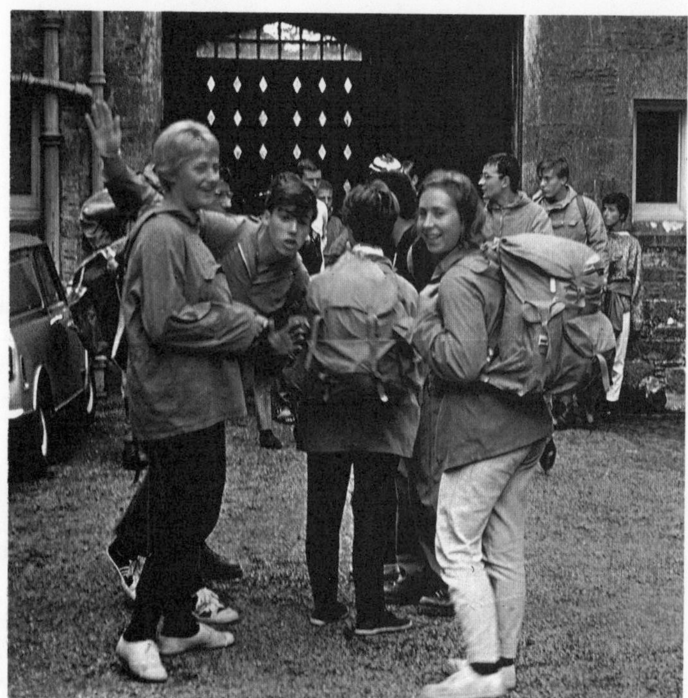

Today's adolescents are on the move far more than previous generations. Many tour this country as well as much of Europe and Asia before going on to higher education. Youth hostels have helped promote friendships and understanding between youths from all countries (*right*) while offering inexpensive lodgings worldwide. Yet another facet of teen behavior is the channeling of energy into sports excellence (*below*) as a way to gain approval. Teams and instruction in most sports proliferate at schools across the country.

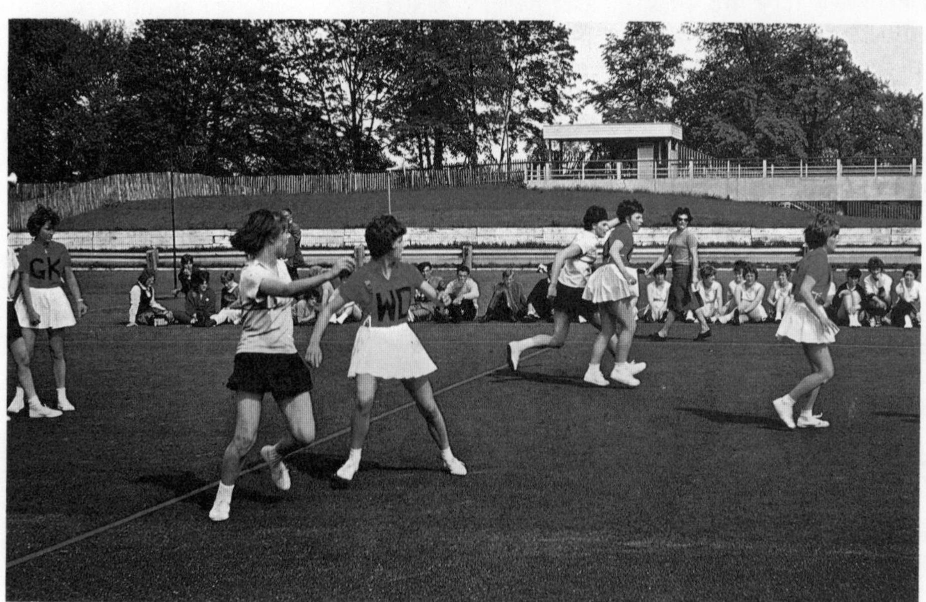


great. It is probable that there are times when adolescents secretly want restraint. They do not *always* want to have all their own way. They are willing to accept the occasional refusal as long as there appear to be good reasons for it, and as long as there has not been too much restraint in the past.

Another source of friction can be the choice of a career. Some teenagers want to leave school or resist going to college, while their parents can see they have the ability to train for a professional career and urge them to remain in school. In other cases, parents interfere too strongly in their children's choices—trying to force them into careers they do not desire or discouraging them from following careers to which they are attracted. The parents have to strike a balance between pushing too hard and doing nothing to guide. Adolescents welcome guidance as long as they do not feel that they are being pushed.

### A MIND OF ONE'S OWN

Adolescents want to think for themselves. Previously all decisions were made for them (by some parents), and now they rebel against this. They rebel against the ways and thoughts of the older generation and may adopt fantastic hair styles and wear unconventional clothes as a sign of their rebellion. This rebellion against tradition may have more serious consequences: sexual license, illegitimate pregnancy, or venereal disease.

By the time adolescents reach college, they have an even greater sense of independence and desire for adult privileges, and have developed strong minds of their own. This accounts for the aggressive behavior of some university students—with their demonstrations and other forms of strident self-assertion.

### LIVE AND LET LIVE

Even when children are adjusting reasonably well to the physical and emotional changes of adolescence and the stresses of their growing independence and responsibilities, a certain amount of friction will exist within the family. The children, especially when they are close in age, develop a keener sense of competition with one another prompted by their newly aroused interest in such areas as sports, physical development, scholastic achievements and the opposite sex. There is apt to be much

**The two photographs below show the contrasting extremes of behavior of which adolescents are capable. Those in the Scout band at left are soberly disciplined as they march, while the two young women at the right work their way into hysteria at the concert of a celebrated rock star.**

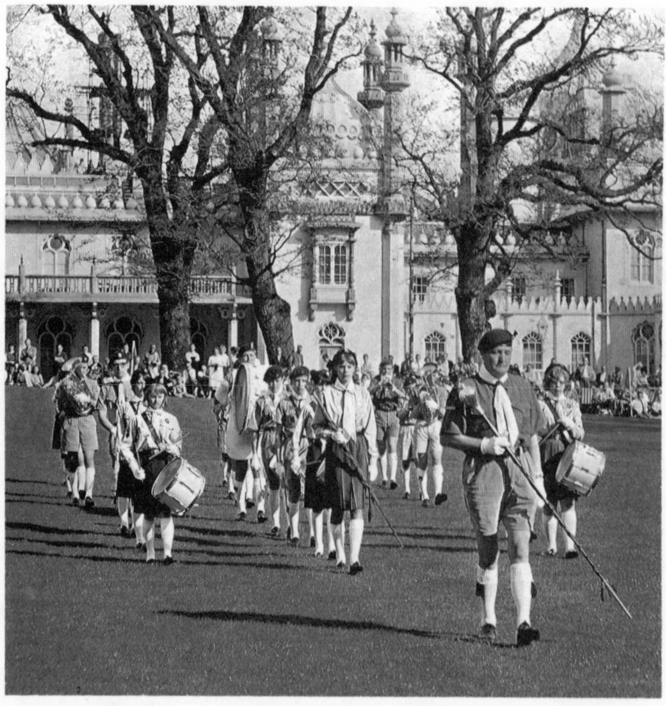

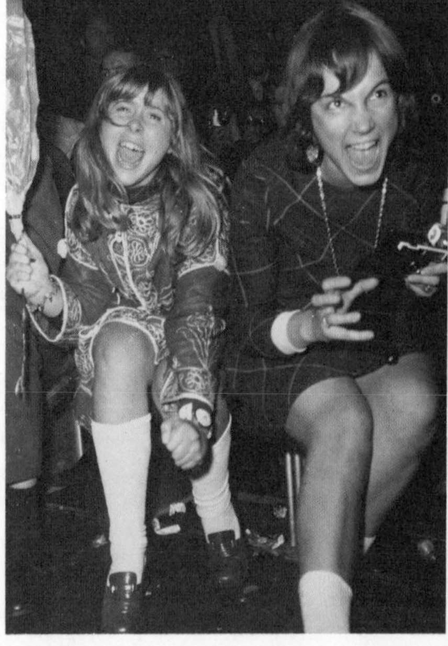

teasing and disparaging banter between them—a lot of it seemingly belligerent. But in stable homes it usually amounts to no more than letting off steam, and for parents it is best to relax and recognize the exchanges for what they are.

Recognition and acceptance by parents of the significance of adolescence in their children's lives is a vital key to the healthy survival of both. The children are becoming adults, in body and mind, and nothing can stop or reverse the process. On the other hand, teenagers still lack the experience that only many more years of living will give them, so they cannot be expected to make mature judgments without help. But help, in the form of parental guidance, cannot avoid all mistakes, and then adolescents need understanding, patience and support. Finally, even the most conscientious parents must accept the fact that though they can love, nurture and train them —and indeed *must* give them standards to live by—they cannot live their children's lives for them.

**ADOPTION** is a satisfying solution to three kinds of problems. First and most important, it gives homeless children a chance to thrive in a relatively normal setting among people who care. It gives another chance to unmarried mothers and to broken families who for various social, financial, or emotional reasons cannot raise their own offspring. It provides an opportunity to would-be parents who have the means, the desire, and the ability to raise children to achieve a fuller family life.

True parenthood is a function of love and care, not of biology. The demand for children is greater than ever. Easier social acceptance of adoption makes it a readier solution for the one in six marriages that is childless because of infertility. A growing number of couples, concerned about rising population, are making the deliberate choice not to have children of their own, or to limit the number drastically, and to adopt children instead. Broadening of eligibility among adoptive parents has encouraged adoption agencies—depending on the particular child and his needs —to place their wards with older couples and even with single women or men.

Some factors have curtailed or altered the supply of adoptable children. Liberalized abortion laws and the widespread use of modern contraceptive devices and drugs by women have sharply decreased the number of babies born out of wedlock. It is also now more socially acceptable for an unmarried mother to keep her baby. Waiting lists for babies are long at all adoption agencies.

More adoptive parents are considering the possibility of adopting an older child. Such children, who may range in age from 2 to 12 years or more, are in greater supply. These may be children who for one reason or another never were adopted as infants and have been kept in institutions or foster homes. Or they may be children under the jurisdiction of the courts, either because their parents have died and no other family placement is at hand or because they have been taken away from broken or seriously disturbed homes. Such children, who have not had happy experiences, may have emotional problems. Some of them may not have been adopted before because of physical or mental deficiencies. A willingness to undertake the parenthood of such children—and the talent to carry it out successfully—requires a rather special kind of adoptive parents who have the patience to wait for, and the ability to earn, the satisfactions of adoptive parenthood.

The many difficulties in adoption should make the prospective adoptive parents weigh carefully the advantages of working with an established licensed agency as opposed to the so-called black market. By-passing the licensed agency may occasionally be the quicker means of getting a baby, but it holds certain hazards. For one, the adoptive parent generally has no knowledge of the biological mother's state of health, nor has the baby been observed medically for a long enough period for birth defects or diseases to be apparent. While some adoptive parents may be ready and willing to love and care for a defective baby or child, most who seek a newborn baby are not prepared to have such defects come as an unwelcome surprise.

The best way to protect an adoption is to negotiate it through an approved and licensed agency. There are no better experts on the legal questions concerning adoption. The adoption agency goes to great lengths to make sure that the children it processes are legally free. Professional social workers have made certain that the biological mother has

**Adoption**—This tot has adapted nicely to her new home. Adoptions using the experience of licensed agencies have more chance for success.

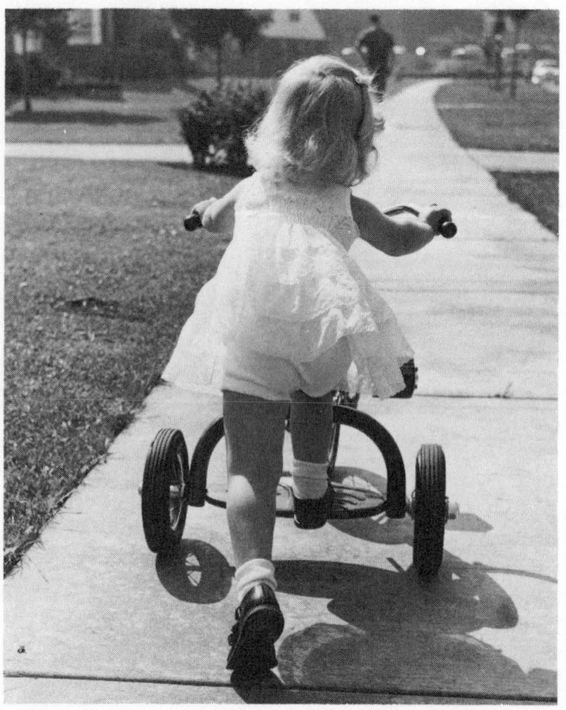

considered all aspects of surrendering her baby and truly wants to do so. The adoption agency will process all the legal papers of surrender and adoption and make sure that they conform to the laws, which vary considerably in these matters from state to state. One can also have greater confidence with a licensed agency that the biologic mother and the baby have been under proper medical supervision and observation for some time.

The likelihood of a successful adoption is greater with a licensed agency because their social workers are experienced at matching children with the proper homes. Children and would-be parents differ widely; it is often a mistake to place an aggressive, overly active child in a fastidious home. The adoption worker's evaluation of the child and of the adoptive parents provides the basis for better security for both.

There are many different types of licensed adoption agencies. Some private ones are affiliated with religious organizations, but there are many nonsectarian agencies as well. In addition, adoption services are provided by state, county, and municipal welfare agencies. All must conform to state laws. Virtually all share lists of children who are hard to place, and they can provide information concerning the adoption of foreign children, if that is the adoptive parents' choice.

A list of licensed adoption agencies can be secured from the State Department of Public Welfare, the local Council of Social Agencies, or from the local Community Chest or United Fund. These are the sources to contact whether the wish is to adopt a child or to surrender one for adoption. These agencies will provide experienced help and advice for unmarried mothers, without reproaches or embarrassment.

After an adoption agency has been contacted and an application for a child has been made, a social worker will come to make a "home study." It is important to understand that the purpose of this is not to pry, and that the professional social worker's scale of values is very broad. It makes little difference to the social worker whether the house is tidy or in disarray, except to the extent that this may provide the clue to the type of child who will thrive there. Nor is the family's income or social status an important factor; there are often funds available to help support a child whose care entails expenses beyond a family's means, provided that the home is right for the child. This is especially true for the hard-to-place child with physical, mental, or emotional handicaps. Care—not money—is the important thing to the agency.

The chief purpose of the social worker's visit is to ascertain the applicant's desire and aptitude to raise an adopted child, and to help determine what kind of child will best fit into that particular home. The motivation for wanting an adopted child will undoubtedly come under discussion, and it would be wise for applicants to know their own minds and motives in this matter. Importantly, husband and wife should agree on wanting the adoption. If both adoptive parents work (or if the single applicant parent works), the social worker will want to be sure that satisfactory arrangements can be made for the daytime care of the child. The applicant who loves children and who is open and natural with the adoption agency should eventually be successful in getting a child *See also* CHILD CARE; FOSTER CHILDREN.

◆ The Child in Society, 80.

**ADRENAL GLAND,** a small triangular gland lying in front and on top of each of the two kidneys. The hormones these glands secrete are essential to life, for among other tasks they regulate the body's metabolism of carbohydrates, fat, and protein, help control the retention of body fluids, and so influence blood pressure, combat the effects of stress and injury, mobilize the body's resources of energy in times of emergency, and influence certain sex characteristics. Loss of the glands—especially of the cortex (outer part)—or of their functions was at one time a virtual sentence of death; but artificial hormones and extracts have overcome this hazard. Some patients who have had both adrenal glands removed (such surgery is sometimes necessary) have been maintained in relatively good health for over 20 years.

Each adrenal has two main parts: *medulla* and *cortex*. Each part has different functions and responds to different stimuli.

The *medulla* (meaning pith or core) is the inner part of the adrenal. Chiefly it produces, stores, and releases at the proper signal the hormones *epinephrine* (also called *adrenalin*) and *norepinephrine* (*noradrenalin*). These are the "fight or flight" hormones that enable the body to rise to emergencies. The medulla is linked with the *sympathetic nervous system,* which signals it to release its hormones in times of danger, fear, anger, or sudden stress. The substances, pumped into the bloodstream, bring about their dramatic effects in seconds. Pupils dilate for better sight, blood pressure rises, the heart beats faster, and breathing is speeded up. The blood vessels near the skin contract so that there will be less loss of blood and faster clotting if wounded. The reactions of the central nervous system are heightened. Most importantly, the medullary hormones cause quick release of reserve stores of glycogen from the liver and provide chemical means for muscles to quicken their conversion of these carbohydrate reserves into energy. So efficient is the system that ordinary people in times of extreme stress have been known to perform feats of extraordinary strength and endurance. Because it re-

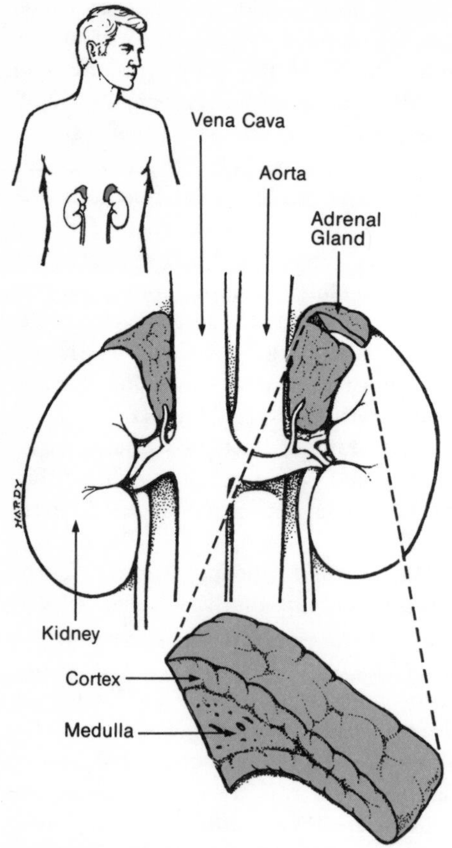


**Adrenal Gland**—The small adrenal gland atop each kidney produces some of the body's most indispensable hormones. The outer shell (cortex), most often interacting with the pituitary gland, releases hormones known as steroids that govern a wide variey of essential actions of metabolism. The inner core (medulla) produces the "fight or flight" hormones that equip the body to cope with emergencies.

laxes bronchial muscles, manufactured epinephrine may be used as a drug to relieve asthma and hay fever.

The *cortex* (meaning bark or rind) is the outer part of the adrenal gland. Almost all of its hormonal production is stimulated by interaction with the *pituitary* gland via the pituitary hormone *ACTH* (*adrenocorticotrophin*). The adrenal cortex is a veritable chemical factory, producing over 30 hormones that carry out a wide variety of metabolic assignments in maintaining body functions in health and disease. These hormones belong to a chemical classification called *steroids.* They are produced by the adrenal cortex and are known as *adrenocorticosteroids.* They are classified into three groups: *mineralocorticoids, glucocorticoids,* and *sex steroids.*

*Mineralocorticoids* control the body's balance of vital mineral substances—in particular, sodium, chloride, and potassium. Sodium chloride (salt) has special importance in that it is the medium by which body water is retained or eliminated and body cells exchange nutrients and by-products. Thus, if the body retains too much salt, it also retains too much water, the tissues swell with edema, and the fluid volume in blood vessels increases to such a point that high blood pressure results. If too much salt is lost, too much water is also lost, with resulting low blood pressure, thickened blood, shrinkage of tissues, and shock. Potassium balance is also important, for potassium is a vital part of the chemistry in which muscles and nerves derive their strength and sensivitity.

The most important of the mineralocorticoids is *aldosterone.* Aldosterone production interacts chiefly with an enzyme called *renin,* which is produced by the kidneys. The kidneys, with their rich blood supply, are immediately sensitive to changes in blood volume; they are the main organs through which body salt and water are retained or eliminated. Aldosterone also affects salt and water retention in sweat and saliva.

*Glucocorticoids*—their production by the adrenals directly stimulated by pituitary ACTH—are among the most essential hormones. They control the way in which the body mobilizes, breaks down, and uses vital energy-providing and body-building substances like carbohydrates, fats, and proteins. The most important and abundant hormone in this group is *cortisol,* also known as *hydro-*

*cortisone.* Of special significance is the ability of the adrenal cortex to produce these substances in increased quantities in times of stress, signaled by increased ACTH. The stress can be of almost any type: physical restraint, injury, intense heat or cold, illness, surgical operations, injection or ingestion of toxic substances.

The glucocorticoids work in yet another protective way by preventing inflammation. Their anti-inflammatory properties enable physicians to use them as drugs in combatting severe arthritis, rheumatic fever, and allergic reactions. In the violent allergic response called *anaphylaxis,* administration of glucocorticoid can be life-saving.

*Sex steroids* produced by the adrenal cortex consist mainly of *androgens,* which determine male sex characteristics. Very small quantities of *progesterone* and *estrogen,* female sex hormones, are also secreted. Normally, the adrenal androgens have very little effect, except perhaps for determining the development of underarm hair in both sexes and pubic hair in females—the more important site of sex hormone production is in the *gonads* (sex glands). However, when adrenal gland production of androgens is abnormally high, marked masculinizing effects occur. *See also* ACHARD-THIERS SYNDROME; ACTH; ADRENAL GLAND DISORDERS; ADRENALIN; ADRENOCORTICAL INSUFFICIENCY; ADRENOGENITAL SYNDROME; ALDOSTERONISM *and* **medigraphs** ADDISON'S DISEASE; CUSHING'S SYNDROME; HYPOGLYCEMIA.

▶ The Endocrine Glands, *Location of Endocrine Glands,* 1047; *The Adrenal Glands,* 1055.

◆ Master Glands of the Human Body, 1370. Controlling the Cell System, 1583.

**ADRENAL GLAND DISORDERS.** When the adrenals are affected by disease, a wide variety of disorders can result, depending on which aspect of adrenal function is affected, to what extent, and in what manner. Generally such disorders are either disorders of underproduction or of overproduction.

DISORDERS OF ADRENAL UNDERPRODUCTION (*Hypoadrenalism*). In these disorders, the life-threatening dangers of adrenal underproduction are related to the cortex. The hormones of the medulla are not essential to life, and under ordinary conditions are secreted in such minute quantities that their absence makes little difference to normal functioning. The hormones of the cortex, however, are essential for the body's normal needs.

Chronic adrenal insufficiency is called *Addison's disease* (after the physician who in 1855 first described what happened when the adrenal glands were destroyed). It affects about one in 100,000 people. Failure of the adrenal glands occurs when the adrenal cortex atrophies (withers away). In about half the cases, the cause is unknown; but in a little less than half, the cause is a fungal or tuberculous infection. In a small number, the condition may be due to infiltration of cancer or leukemia, starchy deposits, or to a blood disorder called *hemochromocytosis.* In some cases, a milder version of the disorder is caused by the failure of the pituitary gland to secrete sufficient ACTH to stimulate the adrenals.

The effects are serious, the degree of gravity depending on how quickly the atrophy is proceeding.

The deficiency of *mineralocorticoids* causes the body to lose salt and potassium. Body water then shrinks, blood volume and pressure fall drastically, blood thickens, and muscles lose responsiveness. The deficiency of *glucocorticoids* makes it impossible for the body to handle carbohydrates, fats, or proteins, and the patient's energy wanes. In addition, the body is vulnerable to inflammation and cannot respond to injury and stress. In some persons with the disease, dark pigmented blotches appear, usually in the thin skin of the lips and nipples and at pressure points of knees, elbows, and knuckles. Early symptoms are loss of weight, easy fatigue, stomach cramps, nausea, diarrhea, and skin pigmentation.

Without treatment, the disease is fatal; the patient will die of shock a few days after the adrenals completely lose function. Fortunately, the onset of the disease is usually slow, its presence can be detected relatively early by modern laboratory techniques, and effective treatment is available. The basis of treatment is the artificial replacement of the adrenal hormones wasted by the disease. The most important of these hormones can now be manufactured or extracted from animals. If the disorder is due to pituitary failure, the physician will administer the missing ACTH. If the cause is primarily in the adrenals, physicians will maintain the patient on artificial mineralocorticoids and glucocorticoids.

If tuberculosis does not cause increased damage to the adrenals, patients with Addison's disease can lead relatively normal lives. The replacement drugs, however, must be taken regularly as long as the patient lives; and frequent checkups are important. Such patients should carry proper identification and be prepared for stressful emergencies, for at such times they need special care and increased doses of their corticosteroids under medical supervision.

DISORDERS OF ADRENAL OVERPRODUCTION (*Hyperadrenalism*). Overproduction of adrenal hormones can be caused by hormone-producing tumors either in the pituitary gland or in the adrenals, or by excessive tissue growth in these glands due to unknown causes. When the fault is in the pituitary, excess ACTH is produced, which overstimulates the adrenal cortex in all its functions. When the fault is primarily in the adrenals, excess production may occur in all the adrenal hormones or just in one or two.

*Cushing's syndrome* is produced when all of the adrenal cortex hormones are overproduced. It is a rare disease seen more frequently in women than in men, usually appearing in the 20's and 30's, particularly after pregnancy. The overproduction of the mineralocorticoids increases salt and water retention, causing some edema and puffiness and from moderate to severe high blood pressure. More serious and evident is the result of glucocorticoid overproduction. The increased carbohydrate metabolism can bring about a diabetic condition by "burning out" the liver cells that help process sugars. Proteins are depleted, wasting away muscles and bones. Fat metabolism is affected so that fat deposits become abnormally distributed, causing a characteristic "buffalo hump" behind the neck and the round, obese "moon face." Overproduction of sex steroids—mostly androgen—can bring about masculinizing effects in women, such as beard growth, deep voice, baldness, and even the extension of the clitoris to penis-like proportions.

Treatment is to try to decrease ACTH adrenal stimulation by destroying the pituitary gland or its tumor with surgery or radiation. If that is not possible, all or part of the adrenals is removed surgically, and if any hormonal insufficiency then develops, artificial steroids are prescribed.

Overproduction of *aldosterone*. is called *primary aldosteronism*. The excess of this mineralocorticoid causes abnormal retention of sodium, chloride, and water; and it brings about abnormal loss of potassium. With increased fluid and blood volume, high blood pressure results. The loss of potassium causes muscle cramps and weakness—even attacks of paralysis. Blood becomes alkaline. The kidneys become damaged because of their inability to process the salt-concentrated urine. Treatment is by surgical removal of the tumor causing the defect, with dramatic improvement.

Overproduction of sex hormones is called *adrenogenital syndrome.* In young children, the cause is commonly congenital overdevelopment—*hyperplasia*—of this portion of the adrenals. There may also be a congenital deficiency of enzymes needed for the production of these hormones. In girls, the result is *virilism,* with the development of external genitals partly male and partly female; the enlarged clitoris can even be mistaken for a penis. If untreated, such girls become broadshouldered, bearded, and without breast development. In boys, the penis grows to adult size in childhood, pubic hair appears by age 4 or 5, and the general body build becomes like that of a man, although such boys are usually short at full growth. Generally, these children also suffer from insufficiency of other adrenal hormones because the androgens are being produced at the expense of glucocorticoids; indeed, this poses the greater danger. Treatment consists of administering cortisol-type hormones, and the resulting hormonal balance usually brings about some correction of the abnormal sexual development. In girls, after the condition has been corrected, plastic surgery of the enlarged genitals can be performed.

Virilization of females and precocious puberty in males may occur when the condition is acquired after childhood. Although excessive sex steroid is almost always the masculinizing androgen, sometimes excess *estrogen*—a feminizing hormone—is secreted in excess in boys and men. The result is shrinkage of the testes, loss of body hair, and breast development. Because the acquired form of adrenogenital syndrome is most commonly a tumor, treatment is surgical, with rapid and dramatic result.

Overproduction of hormones caused by hormone-producing tumors in the

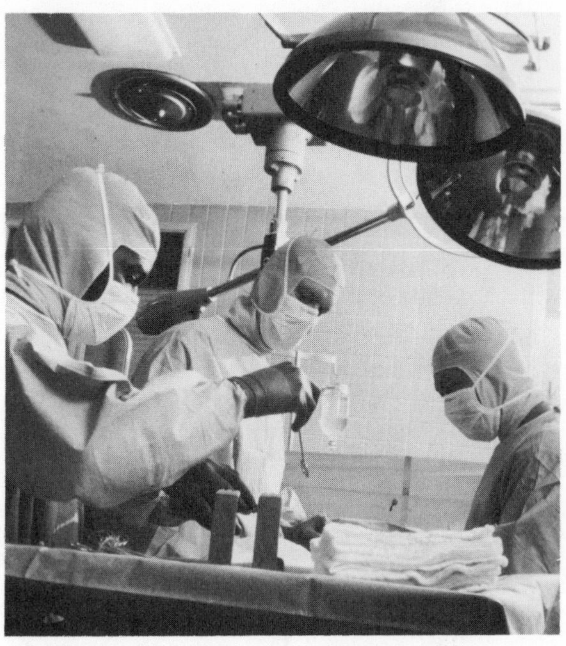

**Adrenal Gland Disorders**—Sometimes surgery is required to correct an adrenal gland problem. Disorders vary, depending on which hormones are produced to excess. With too much aldosterone, for example, there is loss of potassium causing muscle cramps and weakness. Too many sex hormones cause virilization in females and sexual precocity or feminization in males.

*medulla,* or in the cells of its associated sympathetic nervous system, is called *pheochromocytoma.* Because the medullary hormones *epinephrine* and *norepinephrine* are emergency-serving hormones, their overproduction keeps the patient in a continual state of physical alarm, with serious consequences. High blood pressure and increased nervousness are the main results. The symptoms may be continuous or fluctuating with occasional severe attacks. Patients experience pounding headaches, sweating, heart palpitation, trembling, nausea, pain in the chest and abdomen, and prickling sensations in the hands and feet. Neurotic manifestations may appear. The treatment is surgical removal of the tumor. Unless there has been kidney damage because of the high blood pressure, such surgery usually eliminates the symptoms completely. *See also* ACTH; ADRENAL GLAND; ADRENALIN; HYPERADRENALISM; HYPOADRENALISM; VIRILISM *and* **medigraphs** ADDISON'S DISEASE; CUSHING'S SYNDROME.

▶ The Endocrine Glands, *The Adrenal Glands,* 1055. The Importance of Skin, *Skin and Aging,* 2710.

**ADRENALIN,** the trade name for *epinephrine,* the "fight or flight" hormone secreted by the *medulla* portion of the adrenal glands. It speeds up the heart, raises blood pressure, increases oxygen consumption, constricts surface blood vessels, and makes quick energy available to muscles. As a drug, it relaxes bronchial muscles and helps ease asthma. It is also used to counter the effects of severe allergic reactions and overdoses of insulin. *See also* ADRENAL GLAND; ADRENAL GLAND DISORDERS; ALLERGY; ASTHMA.

**ADRENOCORTICAL INSUFFICIENCY,** *hypoadrenalism,* or *Addison's disease,* the disorder caused by underproduction of the hormones in the cortex region of the adrenal glands. As a result, the body's balance of water, salt, and potassium is disturbed, with life-threatening implications when the condition is serious. Also, patients with this disease are unable to metabolize carbohydrates, fats, and proteins properly, and their ability to fight off inflammatory diseases is diminished. *See also* ADRENAL GLAND; ADRENAL GLAND DISORDERS *and* **medigraph** ADDISON'S DISEASE.

**ADRENOCORTICOTROPIC HORMONE.** *See* ACTH.

**ADRENOGENITAL SYNDROME,** a disorder caused by overproduction of sex hormones—mainly *androgens*—in the adrenal glands. The effects are masculinizing; females with the condition may develop deep voices, sprout beards and increased body hair, become bald, have increased muscularity, and the clitoris may enlarge to penis-like proportions. Older males are relatively little affected except in rare cases where the over-secreted substance is *estrogen,* a feminizing hormone, which may bring about breast enlargement. Young boys with the condition, however, develop adult penises, muscles, and sex drives precociously.

The cause is almost always a tumor, and the treatment is to remove the tumor surgically. *See also* ADRENAL GLAND; ADRENAL GLAND DISORDERS; ANDROGEN; ESTROGEN.

▶ The Endocrine Glands, *The Adrenal Glands,* 1055.

**AEDES AEGYPTI,** a species of mosquito living in tropical and subtropical zones, responsible for the transmission of the virus of *yellow fever.* The female mosquito is the carrier. It becomes infected feeding on the blood of a yellow fever patient during the first three or four days of his illness, and is capable for the following 10–12 days of transferring the virus to someone else. *See also* INSECT BITES; MOSQUITO BITES *and* **medigraph** YELLOW FEVER.

**AEROBE,** a microorganism—specifically a *bacterium*—that lives and grows in the presence of oxygen, as opposed to an *anaerobe,* which does not require oxygen for life. The descriptive terms are *aerobic* or *anaerobic.* Aerobic organisms may be *obligate aerobes,* which cannot survive without oxygen; or they may be *faculative aerobes,* which can use oxygen if it is present but can survive by other means in its absence. An aerobe is said to *respire,* in that it emits carbon dioxide as a by-product of its metabolism of oxygen. *See also* BACTERIA.

◆ Bacteria—Agents of Decay, 324.

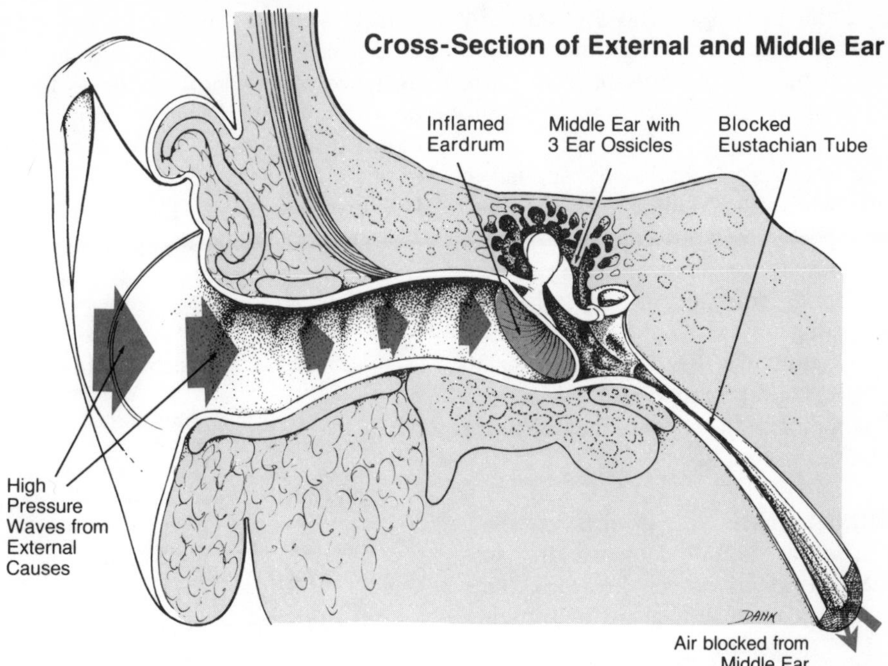


**Aero Otitis Media**—Air pressure on the outside of the eardrum greater than that on the inside causes the eardrum to become inflamed and painful. One type of situation producing this condition is airplane descent when pressurization is insufficient. Clearing the Eustachean tube by yawning or swallowing may bring relief when air from the throat counterbalances eardrum pressure.

**AERO OTITIS MEDIA,** a painful inflammation of the middle ear caused by changes in air pressure. It is a common occurrence in airplanes, the change in pressure being brought about during descent from high altitudes. The condition develops when the pressure against the ear is greater than that from inside, causing the eardrum to bend inward too far. Ordinarily, air in the Eustachian tube, which derives its air from the throat, will counterbalance such pressures and equalize the eardrum so it can vibrate freely. But when the Eustachian tube is blocked—as may happen with a simple cold, ear infection, or allergic condition—painful differences of air pressure on the eardrum can result.

Thus, prevention of the condition consists in keeping open the Eustachian tubes. Air passengers who feel ear pain should yawn heavily, swallow hard, or chew gum to open the tubes. Those who know they are susceptible should use ephedrine-type nose drops or nose sniffers to dry out and open the tubes in advance of and during an air flight, especially if they have a cold. Those with bad colds are well advised to postpone their flights if at all possible.

If the pain persists for any length of time after a flight and is not relieved by simple medicines, a physician should be consulted. *See also* EAR; EAR STUFFINESS; EUSTACHIAN TUBE.

**AEROPHAGIA.** *See* AIR SWALLOWING.

**AEROPHOBIA,** fear of air, exemplified by unrealistic fear of drafts or air in motion. The source of this may go back to long outdated theories that drafts in themselves bring disease, to an obsession about germs in the air, or to an actual fear of body odors from others. Such fears, to one degree or another, are not uncommon in people who are generally reasonable and normal in other ways. Some mentally ill patients believe others are attempting to poison the air around them.

The term aerophobia is also applied to people who are afraid to fly in an airplane. Many persons are courageous about most things as long as they are on the ground, and are not apprehensive about being on the heights of tall buildings or mountains. Psychiatrists and psychologists conduct group therapy sessions and clinics for those who fear airplane flight. *See also* PHOBIAS.

**AEROSOL,** spray can devices in which the solid or liquid contents are suspended in a gas under pressure. This provides a convenient means of spraying a wide range of products, including paints, insecticides, stove cleaners, furniture polish, hair sets, lotions, shaving cream, and even some medications.

Spray cans should be handled with caution, for their dangers are twofold. First, the high pressure in the cans may cause them to explode when heat is applied, the valve or can is defective, or the can is punctured. Second, the gases used as propellants, or the contents of the can, may be inflammable, injurious to the skin, eyes, and lungs, or poisonous when swallowed.

The label on each spray device contains warnings and a list of its particular dangers. These should be read carefully before using. Do not put any spray can on a stove or radiator, and keep it away from direct sunlight. Those cans containing inflammable and toxic materials should be used only in well-ventilated areas, preferably in an air current moving from the user to the can and the object being sprayed. When the can is empty, hold it upside down and release all the gas before throwing it away. Even then, the discarded can should not be incinerated.

Call a doctor or go to the hospital emergency room immediately if there is evidence of poisoning or illness from use of a spray, and bring the can. *See also* DRUG ABUSE; FIRST AID *and* **medigraph** GLUES AND SPRAYS.

◆ A Better Life or Utter Chaos? 148. The Helpful Halogens, 657.

RESEARCH REPORT

**POSSIBLE HAZARD TO HEART FUNCTION FROM AEROSOLS**

Interference with normal heart function is another possible human health hazard of the widespread and indiscriminate use of *aerosol* spray can dispensers, according to studies conducted at the NATIONAL INSTITUTE OF ENVIRONMENTAL HEALTH SCIENCES.

It has already been demonstrated that exposure to *aluminum chloride-hydroxide,* a respirable constituent of almost all deodorant sprays, produces lung damage in laboratory animal subjects. It now appears that some of the *fluorocarbons* (*Freons*) which are the propellant gases and solvents in aerosol sprays also depress certain heart functions, such as the contractility of the normal heart muscle. Toxicity studies indicate some of the chemicals in widespread use may be highly toxic to animals with preexisting heart disease or respiratory imbalance.

While the *acute* toxicity of many of the active ingredients in the spray dispensers has been investigated, a great deal is yet to be learned about their cumulative toxicity. NIH925

**AFFECT,** a term used in psychology to designate the conscious mood, attitude, or emotional tone with which a given person meets experiences. For example, some persons thrust into the center of attention may respond with a general affect of shame, some with pride, some with humility. Those who display no emotional response to a challenge are said to have a lack of affect. *See also* EMOTION; EMOTIONAL DISTURBANCES; MENTAL HEALTH; PSYCHIATRY.

**AFFERENT NERVES,** or *sensory nerves,* carry impulses from the outside world to the central nervous system. These impressions are interpreted as the senses: touch, taste, smell, sight, and hearing. Afferent nerves may be distinguished from *efferent nerves,* which carry signals from the brain to the muscles.

**AFRICAN LYMPHOMA,** medically termed *Burkitt's lymphoma,* a disease found mostly in equatorial regions, although some cases have been reported from other areas. It is characterized by a tumor mass of the jaw involving the salivary glands. A virus is believed responsible. Untreated, African lymphoma is rapidly fatal, with death occurring four to six months after onset of the condition. The usual treatment consists of *x-rays* and *chemotherapy. See also* LYMPHOMA; LYMPHOSARCOMA.

**AFTERBIRTH,** or *placenta,* the tissue delivered from the mother after the birth of the baby. This temporary organ, developing in pregnancy, acts as an intermediary between the mother and the fetus, bringing nourishment from the mother to the fetus and disposing of wastes from the fetus to the mother: all through the umbilical cord. The afterbirth may follow the baby in 10–45 minutes, during which time the uterus contracts to very small size and shears it from the uterus wall. *See also* CHILDBIRTH; UMBILICAL CORD.

◆ Birth of a Child, 608. Fate and the Human Egg, 717. Maternal Home of the Unborn, 2385.

**AFTERPAINS,** abdominal cramps felt after childbirth. These are caused by the contractions of the uterus in attempting to regain its normal size. Resembling labor pains, but not as intense, they may be slight or severe, and they may occur for two or three days after delivery, depending on the individual reactivity and physical state of the mother. Afterpains tend to be stronger in women who have previously borne children. They can be relieved by analgesic (pain-relieving) drugs. *See also* CHILDBIRTH.

**AGALACTIA,** a rare condition, usually painful, in which the mother is entirely unable to produce milk for her infant. The cause may be some abnormality in the milk ducts or nipples of the breasts, but emotional disturbances, infection of the breasts, malnutrition, anemia, and childbearing at too early or advanced an age may be factors. Sometimes, milk flow can be restored with breast pumps, drugs, improved nutrition (especially proteins and vitamins), and by attention to any emotional problems. *See also* BREAST FEEDING.

**AGAMMAGLOBULINEMIA,** an *immunological deficiency syndrome,* a disorder in which the globulins of the blood (which serve to protect the body against infection) are deficient. Some cases occur at birth; others begin at about the ninth month. Victims of this disorder have increased susceptibility to infection and to allergies. Because of repeated infections, they may fail to thrive and develop naturally.

**AGAR,** sometimes called *agar-agar,* a dry gelatinous product extracted from red seaweed. In biological research, it performs as a medium for the culture of bacteria. It also has laxative properties when taken internally. *See also* ALGAE.

**AGGLUTINATION,** the clumping together of bacteria or blood cells in reaction to antagonistic agents (*antibodies*) introduced into the solution. It provides a visible means of testing for the presence of these antibodies. For example, if bacteria of a certain type agglutinate when a patient's serum is added to the solution, this shows that the serum is

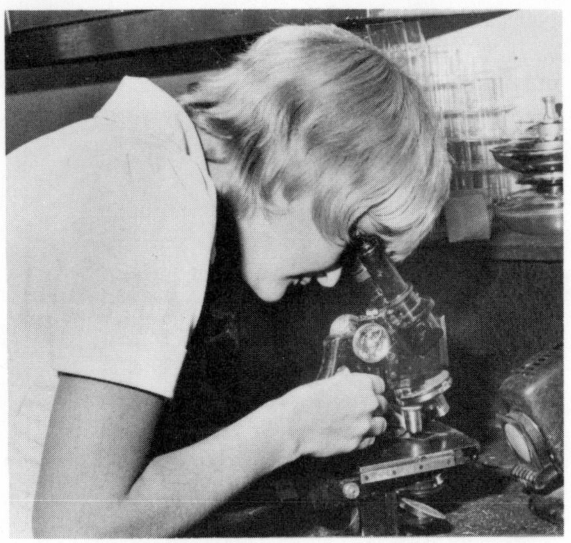

**Agglutination**—A technician observes two blood samples for signs of agglutination—a clumping together of blood cells. It would indicate that the two specimens are not of the same type.

capable of fighting off—or has *immunity* to—that bacteria. In the same way, one can identify and test for the presence of certain organisms by seeing if they agglutinate when an antibody known to be specific to that organism is added. Mismatched blood will agglutinate as in a test for compatibility of blood in blood transfusions. A large number of laboratory tests, many important in diagnosis, are based on this principle.

**AGING.** In 1900, people in North America lived to an average age of about 55; today the life expectancy here is about 71. Medical science and improved public health measures have succeeded in eliminating or curing many diseases that caused early death. The average age at death has stayed between 70 and 72 for many years. Possibly, the only medical advance that will raise it further is the discovery of—and the answer to—the causes of natural aging and death.

Nobody knows for sure why we age and die. Even without illness, nothing can stop the inherent genetic program that patterns our common life history: we grow, we mature, we stop growing, we deteriorate, and eventually we die. In the aging process, sexual appetite wanes and reproductive function ends; cells either shrink or store deposits of fat and calcium; brain cells are lost; starchy deposits called *amyloid* invade the tissues; arteries harden or become blocked; muscles lose resilience; and mechanisms for fighting off disease lose their potency.

While the general format of this life history is the same for everyone, wide differences in its style, length, and speed may occur. Some people lose their full mental capacity early, while others retain their alertness and creativity to old age. Some elderly people of 90 have sexual appetites and vigorous circulation systems despite other signs of aging, while other people only in their 60's lose the sex drive and have hardened arteries. Some skins wrinkle early, some late.

The reasons for variation lie in a combination of genetic and environmental factors. Many people die before their natural time because of life conditions and living habits that accelerate the aging process. In others, the genetic clockwork is so strong, and their inborn constitution so hardy, that they live to very old age despite living conditions and habits that would bring much earlier death to others.

At present, medical science can do little about the genetic program. Treatment with hormones seems to have brought more vigor into some elderly patients' lives, but whether or not this treatment can actually slow the clock is debatable. Some researchers have begun recently to study how to control the deposits of amyloid, hoping that this will provide an important key to one of the physiological processes of aging. Others are seeking ways of strengthening the aging immunological system. Some are concentrating on the *collagen* (connective) *tissues,* in the belief that this is the

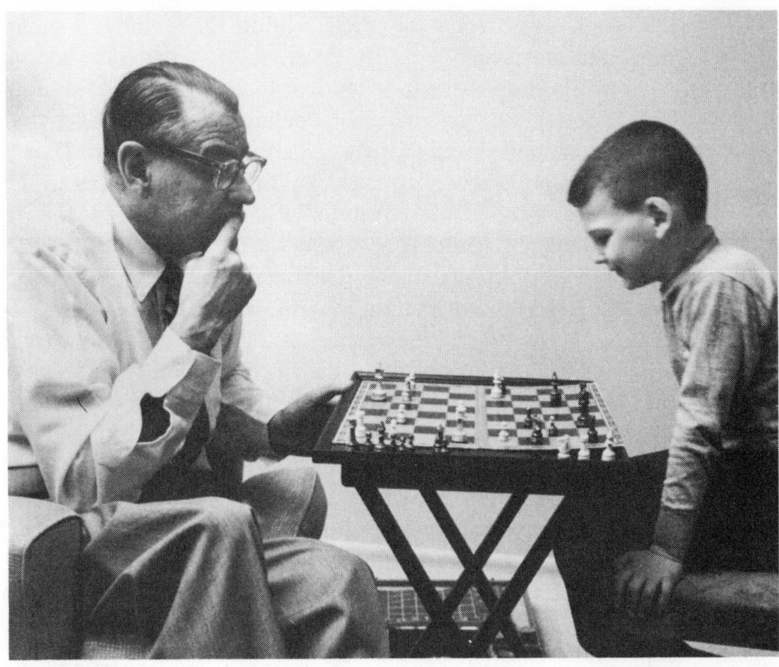

**Aging**—The challenge of chess games with his grandson keeps this retired man mentally active. Pursuit of such special interests is one key to a healthy old age.

central factor. However, how we live may help determine how long we live.

*Physical activity* is important. Very old people have usually led physically active lives and have kept themselves in good physical shape. Muscles, heart, arteries, and lungs all have the capability of losing function when not used to capacity. Only by physical activity are the heart, lungs, and circulation kept in tone so that they can do their vital work of bringing nutrition and healing to all tissues and be prepared to withstand the sudden strains of emergencies. People in sedentary occupations and retired people may keep themselves in trim with daily calisthenics, frequent walking, and with such sports as golf, swimming, or bicycling. The improved sense of well-being that comes from exercise is also important.

*Psychologic and emotional factors* influence the length of life and the quality of aging. People who maintain a positive attitude toward life, remain curious and mentally active, and are emotionally secure generally live longer.

The brain, like muscle, thrives on use and deteriorates when not used. This is so even though all people, after a certain age, undergo a gradual loss of brain cells. This organic change is faster in some than in others, producing loss of memory and sometimes even a changed behavior that in its extreme form is diagnosed as *senile dementia.* In some persons the organic process is so strong that senile dementia occurs even under the best of conditions, but others seem to be able to delay it or compensate for it by compelling themselves to remain alert and mentally active—or because they are surrounded by loving and sympathetic people who keep them alert.

The organic personality changes occurring in old age are strongly affected by loneliness and insecurity. When families were larger, lived together, and were more stable, the aged usually had more useful things to do and were surrounded by family members of all ages and by long-time neighbors. They belonged, felt needed, and had a strong emotional bond to life. Aged people do not generally live with their children now, and are forced to retire from active work while still vigorous. They live today in a society on the move. Loneliness, depression, and emotional insecurity are common among today's elderly, and they are less resistant to the effects of organic brain damage. While it is essential for elderly people to arm themselves against this by seeking entertaining, useful, and stimulating activities, few can do this alone. Their children and their communities must find ways of keeping in touch, using them, and making them feel wanted.

*Diet* is another factor in longevity. Thin people generally live longer than fat people. Excess weight taxes the heart and circulation, promotes inactivity, and is usually associated with eating—or insufficiently metabolizing—foods that have a deleterious effect. Some people seem to be able to eat anything and not gain weight, but those with a tendency toward gaining weight must learn to cut down their consumption of food if they wish to lengthen life and have more vigor in old age. Fatty food especially must be avoided by elderly people; these contain *cholesterol,* which may cause clogged veins and arteries.

Most doctors are convinced that *smoking*—especially the inhaling of cigarette smoke—directly affects the length of life. Smoking limits lung capacity (which is essential for circulation) and promotes such life-limiting diseases as lung cancer, emphysema, and heart disease. *See also* GERIATRICS; MIDDLE AGE CHANGE AND PROBLEMS *and* **medigraph** MENOPAUSE.
▶ Planning the Diet, *Problem Areas Relating to Diet for Good Nutrition,* 898. The Human Eye, *Cataracts,* 1163; *Diseases of the Retina,* 1173. The Health of Women, *Disabilities of the Aging Woman,* 1429. The Rheumatic Diseases, *Degenerative Joint Disease,* 2588. The Importance of Skin, *Skin and Weather,* 2689; *Skin and Aging,* 2710. Vision Impairment, *Blindness,* 2946.
◆ The Needs of the Aged, 1343. Why Do We Grow Old? 1362.

RESEARCH REPORT

PARTICIPATION IN THE DECISION IMPORTANT IN RELOCATON OF ELDERLY

Elderly people who have a definite say in the decision to enter *residential care* facilities seem to adjust *far more* successfully to the move than those whose feelings about relocation are not taken into consideration. This conclusion is the result of gerontological research sponsored by the NATIONAL INSTITUTE OF CHILD HEALTH AND HUMAN DEVELOPMENT. It supports the theory that there is a direct relationship between the physical and emotional well-being of older people who enter nursing homes and similar facilities and their autonomous decision to do so.

Those people whose adjustment to the relocation was easier also involved themselves in more activities than those who were not consulted about making the change. NIH1125

## AGING

NATHAN W. SHOCK, PH.D.

ALMOST EVERYONE WISHES to have a long life but no one wants to grow old. This fear and rejection of old age is the result of many misconceptions about aging and the presumption that with aging the development of chronic diseases is inevitable. Research has shown that this commonly held belief is not true. Aging is a normal process associated with living. It is as much a part of the total life pattern as is child-

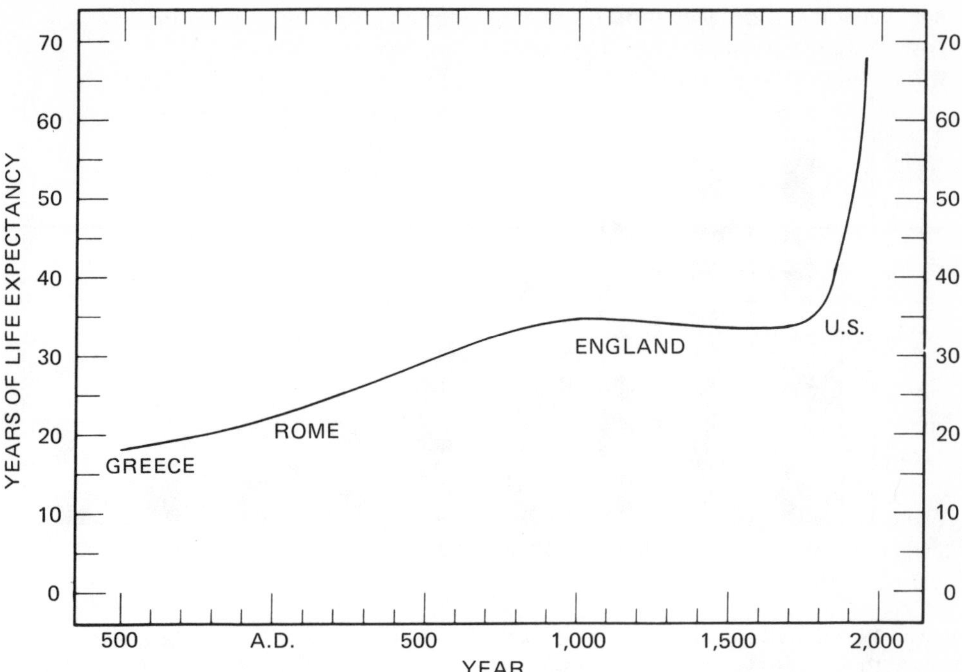


**Fig. 1**—A life expectancy chart shows little improvement from ancient Greece to eighteenth century England but a dramatic rise since then in the United States—to almost 70 years by 1950.

hood and adolescence. It represents the normal changes in physiological characteristics which take place with the passage of time. While it is true that the incidence of many diseases, such as heart disease, cancer, and stroke, increase with age, disease processes may occur at any age. The higher incidence among older people is a reflection that they have lived longer and therefore have had more time for these slowly progressing diseases to develop. Furthermore, many older people do not develop these diseases at all. In fact, only about 5 percent of the population aged 65 and above require nursing home or hospital care. Most elderly people are able to continue to pursue useful and productive lives within the community in spite of the reductions in physiological capacities associated with aging. Advances in medical science have now made possible diagnosis and treatment of many of the chronic diseases which in the past have produced disabilities and impairments among older people.

Historically, the desire for a long life without senescence led to quests for the Fountain of Youth, which were as unsuccessful as current attempts to prolong life with various treatments and nostrums. In the early part of this century claims were made that the injection of extracts made from sex glands or the transplantation of sex glands from young men to older men would result in rejuvenation. Research has shown that none of these procedures will produce any lasting effects and, in fact, may be actually dangerous. Currently, in Europe claims are made that the injection of cells from fetal animals will induce rejuvenation in both men and women, as in the Niehans method. It is also claimed that injections of procaine (Gerovital), as in the Aslan method, will delay or even reverse the progressive effects of aging. None of these claims have been substantiated by carefully controlled experiments.

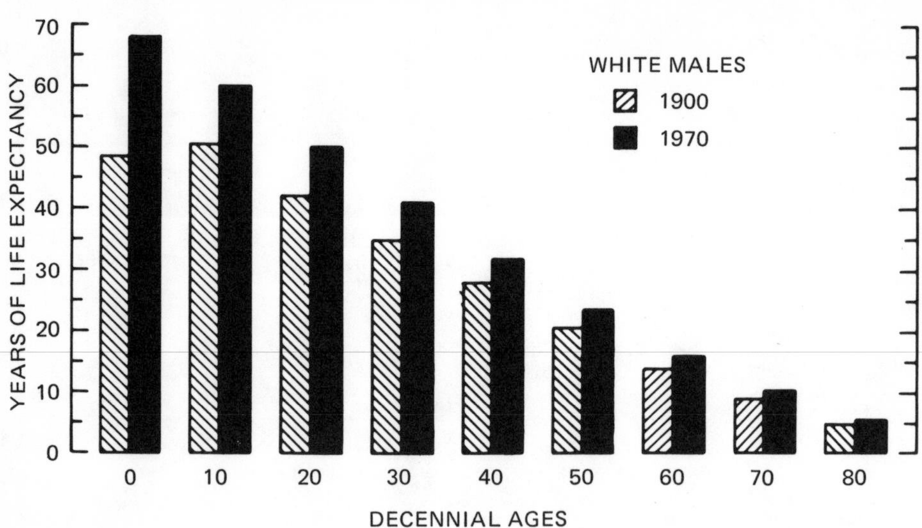


**Fig. 2**—A graph based on data from the Department of Health, Education and Welfare compares remaining life expectancy at each decade for white males in the United States in 1900 and 1970.

## LIFE SPAN

At present the maximum life span that can be validated with evidence of birth dates is about 110–115 years in the human. Claims are made that some individuals can be found who are 130–140 years old. For example, it is claimed that some individuals living in the mountainous area of Georgia in the Soviet Union and in Vilcabamba, Ecuador, and other isolated areas have attained ages of 150–160 years. The great longevity of these people has been ascribed to the fact that they must work hard and maintain a high level of physical activity and that their diets consist largely of grain, vegetables, goat milk, and cheese, with a relatively low intake of meat, cholesterol, and refined sugar. Although many of these people are undoubtedly very old, the absence of adequate birth records makes it impossible to prove their alleged longevity.

The maximum human life span has not changed much over the past 200–300 years. The average age of death, or life expectancy at birth, has increased substantially over the past 100 years. According to the best available estimates from the year 1000 to the late 1800's, life expectancy at birth was about 35 years. However, between 1880 and 1970 in the United States (Fig. 1) life expectancy at birth increased sharply to about 68 years for men and 75 years for women. This increase in life expectancy has also occurred in most other industrialized nations of the world. The highest values of 71 years for men and 76.4 years for women are found in the Netherlands.

In developing countries life expectancy at birth is substantially less than in industrialized societies. For example, in India (1960) life expectancy at birth was 41.9 years in men and 40.6 in women. In Indonesia the comparable values were 47.5 years for both men and women, and in Chile 54.4 years for men and 60 years for women.

Life expectancy is greatly influenced by living conditions, diet, housing, and income levels, as well as the level of medical care available to a population.

Most of the increase in life expectancy at birth between 1900 and 1970 has been the result of the remarkable reduction in infant mortality rates that has occurred over the past 70 years. Actually, the years of life remaining after age 65 has increased very little over the same period. Figure 2 compares years of life remaining at each decade for white men in the United States in 1900 and in 1970. With increasing age, the difference between life expectancies in 1900 and 1970 fall progressively so that men who reach the age of 65 in 1970 can be expected, on the average, to live an additional 13 years. This is only 1.5 years more than the expectancy of men who reached age 65 in 1900.

On the average, women live longer than men. In the United States this sex difference in longevity has been increasing since 1900, when women lived only about 2 years longer than men, to 1970 when the average difference between life span of men and women was approximately 7 years (Fig. 3). Furthermore, death rates for

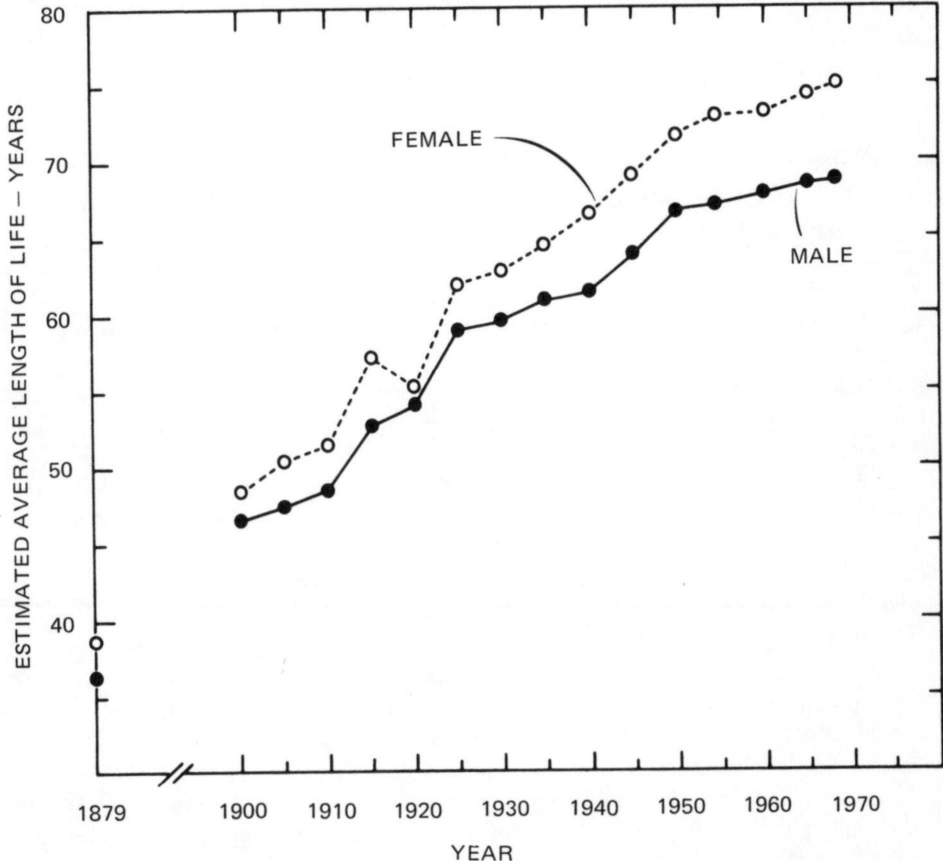


**Fig. 3**—The life spans of women and men in the United States traced from 1900 to 1969 show a consistently longer life for women. It is interesting to note that though the difference increased in the early part of the century, the female life span dropped noticeably in the early 1920's, while the male life span continued a gradual growth. Female length of life rose sharply later that decade, however, and there has been a steady widening of the difference in female/male longevity.

**TABLE 1**
**DEATH RATES IN MALES AND FEMALES BY AGE GROUPS (USA)**

| Age Group | Deaths per 1,000 population in Specified Group | |
|---|---|---|
| | Male | Female |
| Under 1 year | 17.8 | 13.7 |
| 1–4 years | 0.8 | 0.6 |
| 5–14 years | 0.5 | 0.3 |
| 15–24 years | 1.7 | 0.6 |
| 25–34 years | 1.8 | 0.8 |
| 35–44 years | 3.2 | 1.8 |
| 45–54 years | 8.7 | 4.4 |
| 55–59 years | 17.0 | 8.0 |
| 60–64 years | 26.3 | 12.0 |
| 65–69 years | 40.3 | 19.5 |
| 70–74 years | 59.0 | 30.3 |
| 75–79 years | 86.9 | 51.2 |
| 80–84 years | 128.0 | 87.6 |
| 85 years and over | 184.2 | 157.9 |
| Still-births | 16.3 | 14.7 |

Compiled from *Monthly Vital Statistics Report,* National Center for Health Statistics.

men are higher than those for women at every age (Table 1). At age 45–54 there are 8.7 deaths per 1000 men and 4.4 per 1000 women. At age 60–64 the values are 26.3 for men and 12.0 for women. At 75–79 the values are 86.9 for men and 51.2 for women. Even before birth, women have an advantage over men; there are 16.3 male stillborns per 1000 live births compared with 14.7 female stillbirths.

The reason for the increased longevity of women compared with men is not known. Part of the sex difference in total mortality may be due to the greater exposure of men to occupational hazards and accidents. However, it has been found that females of most animal species live longer than males. Female houseflies, rats, mice, dogs and horses, for example, live longer than males when maintained in the same protected laboratory environments. It is therefore assumed that some basic biological characteristic associated with femaleness is associated with increased vitality and longevity. The critical issue is whether the sex difference in vitality is related to the genetic characteristics that determine sex or to the hormones generated by the female sex glands, as for example, estrogens and progesterone, which are produced by the ovary.

Physiologically, females undergo cyclical variations in blood levels of estrogen and progesterone with each menstrual cycle between menarche and the menopause. At the menopause, egg production ceases and the secretion of sex hormones falls so that by age 60 blood levels of female sex hormones in human females is only about 10 percent of the levels observed in young menstruating females. The full physiological significance of the reduction in production of female sex hormones is not understood, but it is at this age that average blood pressure becomes higher in females than in males and the age at which the prevalence of cardiovascular disease in females approaches that found in males.

Although women visit physicians more frequently than men, are hospitalized more frequently, and have more days of restricted activity throughout their entire lives, they live longer than men. For example, 63 percent of the male population age 45–64 reported one or more visits to the physician's office per year as compared with 70.8

**TABLE 2**
**DISABILITY AND UTILIZATION OF HEALTH RESOURCES**

| | Age | Males | Females |
|---|---|---|---|
| Percentage of population visiting physicians one or more times per year | 45–64 years<br>65 + | 63.7%<br>68.1 | 70.8%<br>73.6 |
| Physician visits per year | 45–64 years<br>65 + | 4.1<br>5.5 | 5.2<br>6.6 |
| Hospital discharges per 1000 population | 45–64 years<br>65 + | 143.0<br>254.4 | 160.3<br>237.2 |
| Days of restricted activity per year | 45–64 years<br>65 + | 19.8<br>31.7 | 20.9<br>36.2 |
| Bed disability days | 45–64 years<br>65 + | 7.3<br>12.7 | 7.9<br>14.4 |

From *Health in the Later Years of Life.* U. S. Department of Health, Education, and Welfare, National Center for Health Statistics.

percent of the females (Table 2). In 1970 in the United States the rate of hospital discharges per 1000 population was 143 for men and 160 for women aged 45–64. However, it cannot be assumed that the greater use of health resources by women indicates that their health status is inferior to that of men. It may be argued that increased life expectancy in the female is a reflection of her willingness to seek and utilize medical resources when needed.

The sex difference in mortality produces an excess of women over men in the population which reaches a ratio of 156 women to 100 men at age 75 and above (Table 3). At age 45–64 there are only 109 women per 100 men and at age 65 and over the ratio is 138 women per 100 men. Furthermore, the ratio of women to men in the population over age 65 has been increasing steadily from 111.5 in 1950 to 120.7 in 1960 and 138.5 in 1970. This change in the sex ratio influences the marital status of older men and women. In 1970 64.4 percent of the men over age 65 were married and living with a spouse in contrast to only 33.7 percent of the women. Only 18 percent of the men were widowed in comparison to 54.6 percent of the women aged 65 and over. Since the average age of death is continuing to rise in women whereas there has been only a small increase since 1960 in men (see Fig. 2), the proportion of women in the older population will probably continue to rise.

**TABLE 3**
**SEX RATIO IN THE POPULATION BY AGE GROUPS**

| Women per 100 Men | | Older Women per 100 Older Men (65 +) | |
|---|---|---|---|
| Under 25 years | 98.4 | 1950 | 111.5 |
| 25–44 years | 104.7 | 1960 | 120.7 |
| 45–64 years | 109.1 | 1970 | 138.5 |
| 65 + years | 138.5 | | |
| 65–74 years | 128.8 | | |
| 75 + years | 156.2 | | |

Compiled from *Facts & Figures on Older Americans, #5.* U. S. Department of Health, Education, and Welfare, Administration on Aging.

# PHYSIOLOGICAL AGING

Physiologically, aging is characterized by slow and gradual decrease in the performance capacities of many of the organs of the body. On the average, these changes may begin as early as age 30. However, most of these decrements are so small that they cannot be detected unless the measurements are made at intervals of 20 or more years. A gradual reduction in the amount of blood pumped by the heart, amounting to about a 50 percent decrease between the ages of 30 and 90, could be demonstrated, but the difference between average values for 30- and 40-year-olds was not significant. Furthermore, all data which are available fail to show any rapid loss of function beginning at any specific age, as for example, age 65. This means that aging is a slow and gradual process which extends over the entire life span and a specific age cannot be set as the beginning of senescence or old age. There is no physiological or functional basis for specifying age 65 or 70 as a time for mandatory retirement. On the average, 66-year-old people are not detectably different from 64-year-olds with respect to their physiological characteristics. A retirement age of 65 has been set by custom and cannot be defended on the basis of physiological changes.

A number of physiological functions show a gradual decrement that extends over the entire life span. Visible evidence of aging, such as wrinkling and sagging of the skin, as well as loss and graying of the hair, greatly influences judgments about the age of an individual. These changes in the skin are due primarily to a gradual loss in elasticity. Like old rubber bands, old skin is less likely to return to its original state after being stretched than is young skin. This elastic property is due to the presence of substances called collagen and elastin in the tissue. Laboratory studies have shown that the elastic properties of a tissue are due to the structure of the collagen molecule, which consists of two molecular strands intertwined in a spiral. With increasing age, chemical bonds, called cross-links, develop both between the two strands of one molecule of collagen and also between adjacent molecules. These cross-links greatly reduce the elastic properties of the collagen. These cross-links, which are extremely difficult to break, are believed to accumulate with advancing age. Considerable research is under way to define the factors involved in the formation of cross-links, hopefully to devise methods to reduce their rate of formation and thus to reduce the rate of aging of collagen.

## SENSE ORGANS

Some physiological decrements become apparent to the aging individual. Among these are losses in sensory functions, especially vision and hearing. Old people do not see or hear as well as the young. Visual acuity diminishes so that by age 70, without glasses, poor vision is the rule rather than the exception. The ability to focus the eye on nearer objects falls off. However, most of this change occurs between the ages of 20 and 50 with little change thereafter. Hence it is at the age of 50 that bifocals become necessary. Fortunately, both of these impairments can readily be corrected by appropriate glasses. Similarly, age changes in the lens of the eye may result in opacities and cataracts. Improvements in surgical techniques make it possible to correct these deficiencies when they occur, even at advanced ages. Traditionally, glaucoma has also been a disease of the eye which impairs vision and may ultimately lead to blindness in the elderly. Glaucoma is characterized by a progressive increase of pressure within the eyeball which ultimately damages the retina. New drugs have

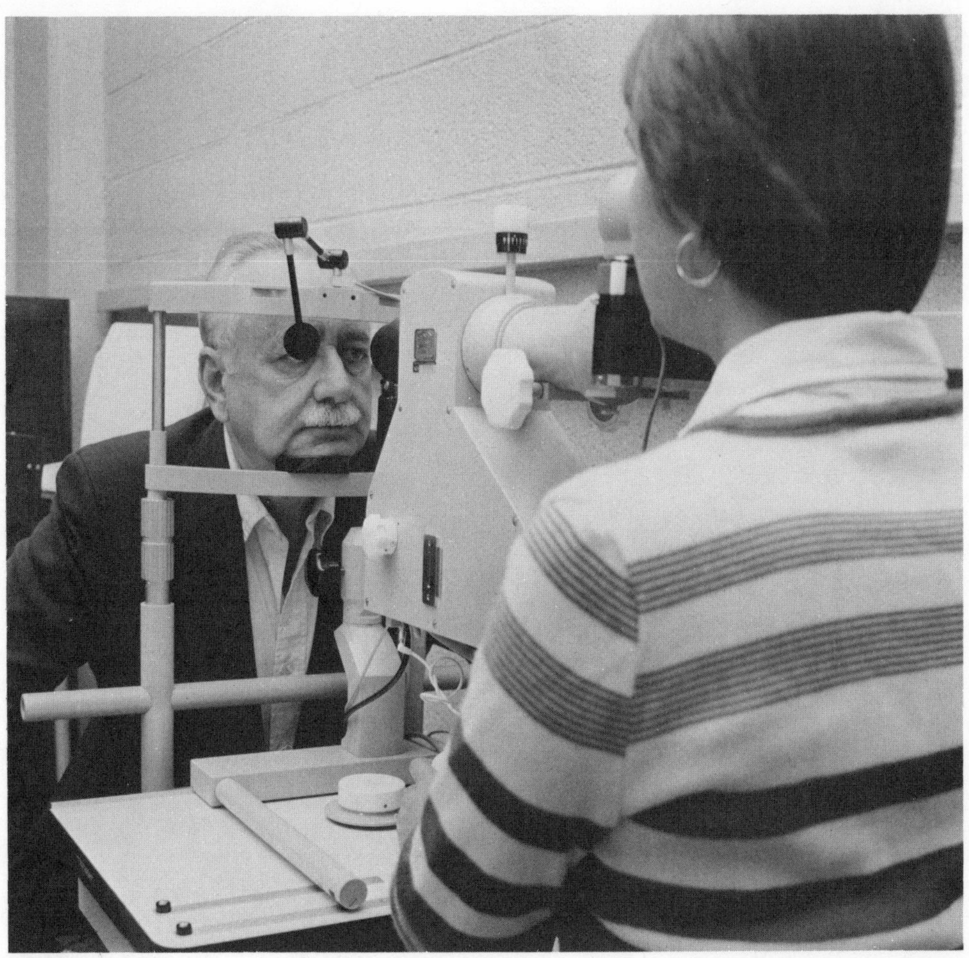

Regular eye examinations not only detect vision problems and the health of the eyes, they are also a window into the body's blood vessel system. The photograph being taken of the man's retina at the back of the eye will reveal the effects of aging on the tiny blood vessels there. In no other part of the body can the complex vascular system be studied while it functions.

been discovered which can control the rise in pressure and can greatly reduce the probability of blindness, providing the disease is detected early. Diagnosis of glaucoma is easily made by measuring the pressure inside the eyeball. This innocuous measurement can be carried out by the ophthalmologist when periodic tests of vision are performed.

With advancing age hearing losses may also occur, especially for high-pitched sounds. Since these tones are important in understanding speech, especially in situations where a number of people are talking at the same time, this sensory loss may have important behavioral implications. However, this age deficit is now correctable through the use of electronic hearing aids.

Recent studies suggest that hearing losses in the elderly may be due to exposure to noise in the environment rather than to inevitable age changes in the ear. A num-

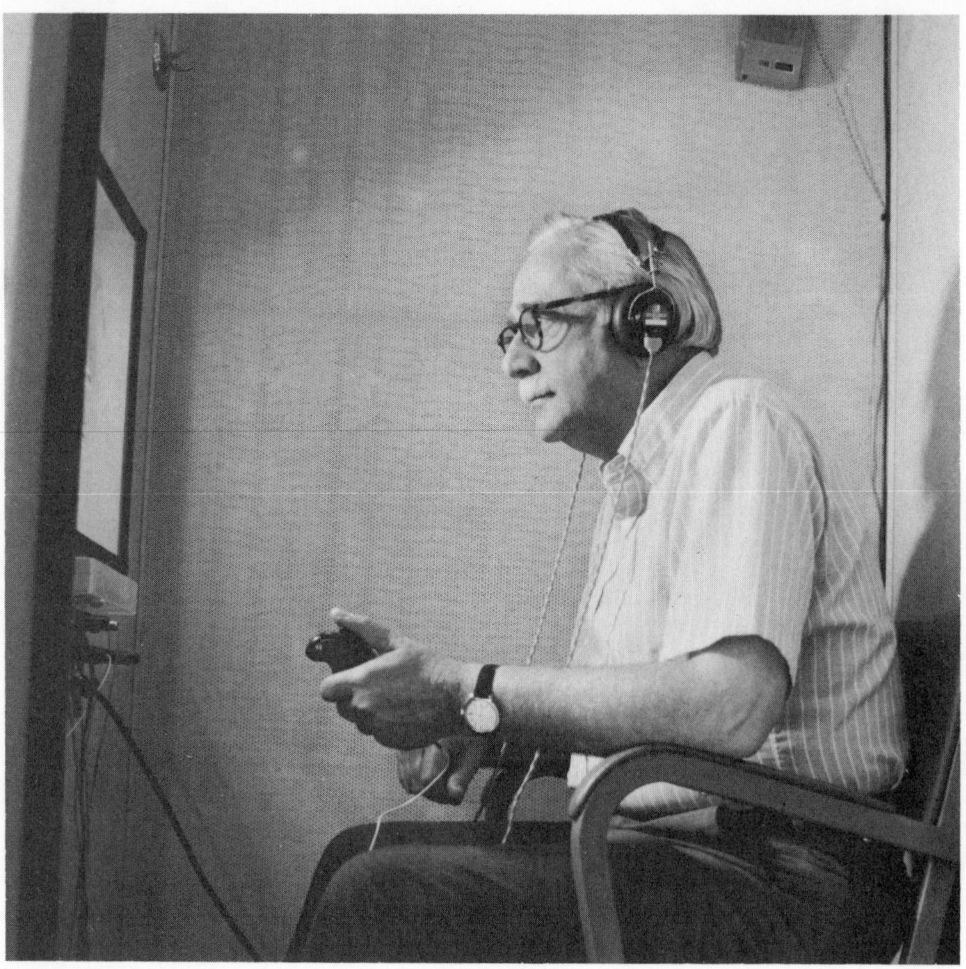

Another sensory function often diminished in the aging process is that of hearing, especially of high-pitched sounds. There are many tests that determine the precise degree of hearing loss. In the test above, as tones of varying pitch and duration are piped into the man's earphones, he presses a button to indicate the levels at which he can no longer hear the tones.

ber of studies have shown that people living in environments where the noise level is low fail to show the age decrements in hearing ability found in people who live in cities of highly industrialized countries. At least a part of the problem of hearing losses is environmental.

Other senses also show age decrements. Sensitivity to taste, especially for sweetness, diminishes after the age of 50. Clinical reports often claim that old people are less sensitive to odors than are the young. Because of the difficulties in separating taste and smell, and the technical difficulties in measuring response to odors, there are no reliable laboratory studies that clearly demonstrate age decrements in sensitivity to odors. However, the sensitivity to taste and smell is influenced by many factors other than age. For example, smoking may play a greater role in impairing these sense modalities than age alone.

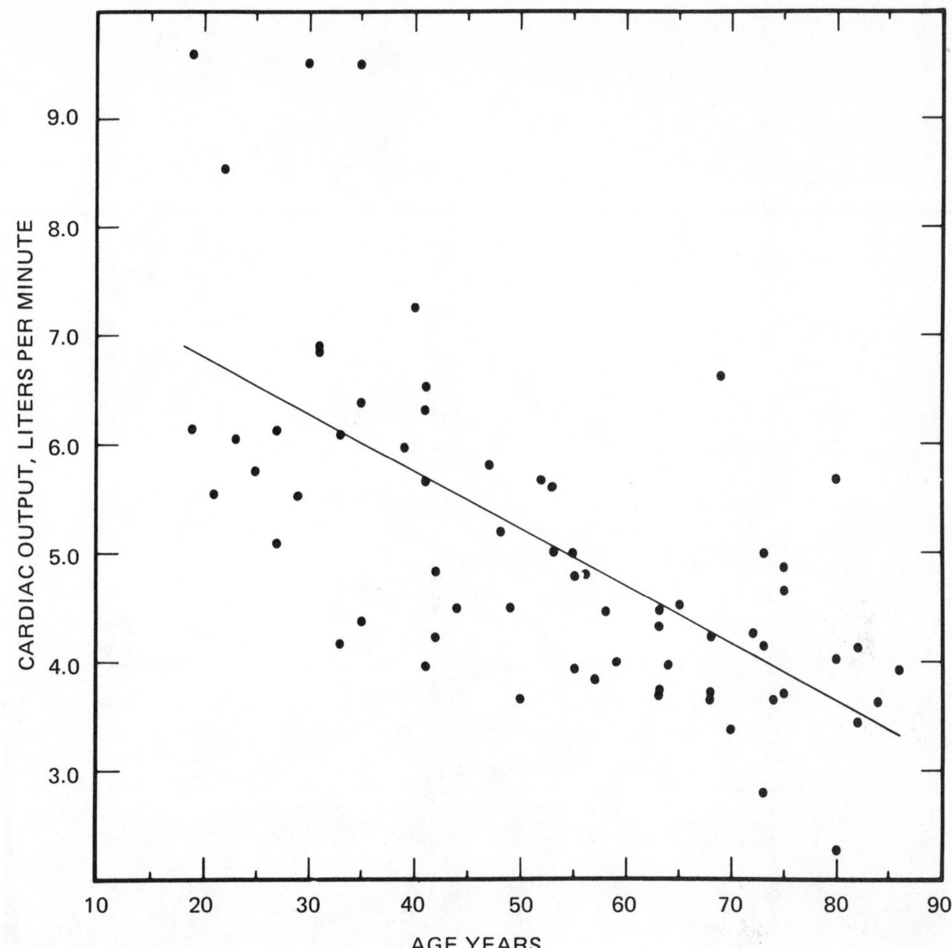


**Fig. 4**—Cardiac output refers to the amount of blood pumped by the heart in a given length of time. The graph above is the result of a test of 67 men, all without a circulatory problem. It demonstrates that cardiac output generally decreases with age but that it is possible at 70 to have pumping action far stronger than some people have in their thirties and forties. Note the wide variance in heart performance among some of those in their twenties, thirties and forties.

Evidence with respect to the effect of age on sensitivity to pain is conflicting. Physicians who deal with aged patients report the impression that the aged are less sensitive to pain than are the young. However, laboratory experiments often fail to show age differences. Part of this discrepancy is because of the difficulties in measuring pain. One laboratory method is to direct radiant heat from a lamp to a part of the body. As the intensity of the light (and heat applied) is gradually increased, the person is asked to indicate when the stimulus becomes painful. He must thus distinguish between the sensation of warmth and of pain. There are individual differences in the ability of people to make this judgment, so it is little wonder that some investigators have reported a reduction in sensitivity to pain in older subjects while others have reported no age differences. Response to pain is a highly individual matter and may be influenced more by personality and cultural factors than by age.

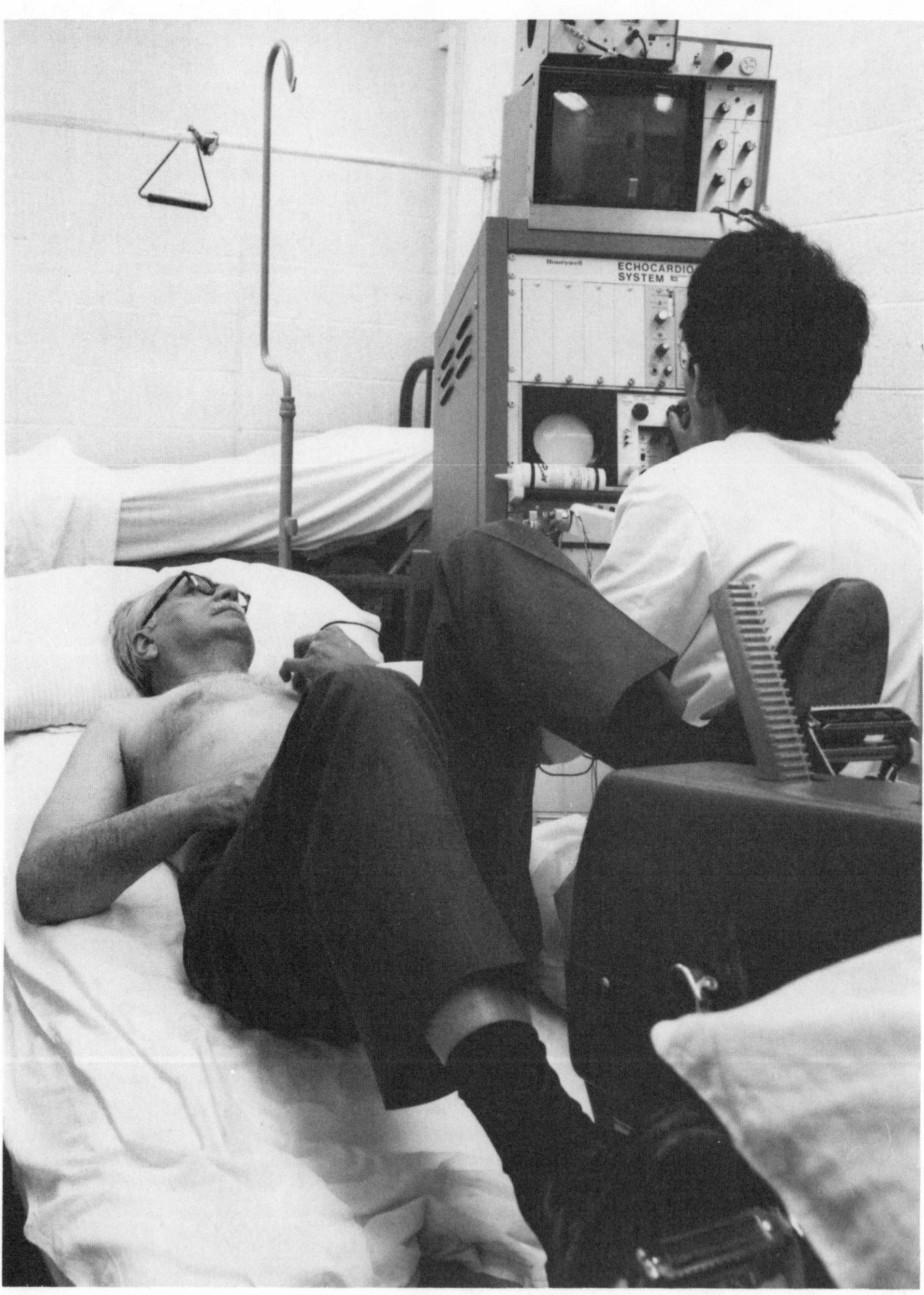


As with the other muscles of the body, the heart ages, too. As it becomes less strong, it pumps less blood and body tissues receive less nourishment. One of the methods doctors use to study an individual's heart performance as it ages is echocardiography, a procedure in which the skin is not punctured nor does an instrument enter the body. Instead, high-frequency sound waves (ultrasound) are beamed into the chest. The various parts of the heart deflect the sound waves and send echoes to a receiver, which records them on moving paper. Variations of heart movement as small as 0.04 inch (1 mm) are revealed by the echoes and become readable on the printout.

In summary, at advanced ages sensory inputs are probably diminished, but the decrements, especially with respect to vision and hearing, can be minimized by the use of glasses and hearing aids.

### AGING OF THE HEART AND BLOOD VESSELS

In order to function properly, every organ and cell of the body must receive an adequate supply of oxygen and nutrients and waste products must be removed. These functions depend on the delivery of blood to the organ and tissues, so that performance of the heart and blood vessels plays a major role in the maintenance of life.

Even in the absence of detectable heart disease, performance of the heart diminishes with advancing age. The amount of blood pumped by the heart under resting conditions falls from an average of 6.5 liters per minute at age 20 to 3.5 liters per minute at age 85 (Fig. 4). Although average values fall with advancing age, differences are found between individuals of the same chronological age (Fig. 5). Thus one 80-year-old subject had a cardiac output of 5.5 liters per minute, which was as good as the average 50-year-old. This wide range of individual differences is characteristic of all physiological measurements so that aging must be regarded as highly individualistic. Chronological age alone is a poor predictor of physiological status of a person.

Structural changes in the heart include a gradual loss of muscle fibers with infiltration of connective tissue. There is a gradual accumulation of insoluble granular material (lipofuscin or "age pigment") in cardiac muscle fibers. These granules, composed of protein and lipids (fats) begin to appear as early as age 20. The amount of pigment gradually increases so that by age 80 the particles may occupy as much as 5–10 percent of the volume of a muscle fiber.

The resting heart rate does not change significantly with age. However, during each beat the muscle fibers of the heart do not contract as quickly in the old as in the young. This reduction in power, or rate of work produced by the heart, is due to a reduction in the activity of certain cellular enzymes that produce the energy for muscle contraction.

On the average, old hearts do not perform as effectively as young hearts, especially when extra demands are made. However, the impairments that can be ascribed to aging are less than those which result from diseases that affect the heart. Consequently, heart failure in the elderly is more apt to be the result of disease than of aging alone.

The incidence of arteriosclerosis (hardening of the arteries) increases with age, and is often regarded as part of aging. This is not necessarily true since the disease may occur at any age. It is a progressive disorder so that by middle age practically everyone has the disease to some extent. However, presence of the disease may not result in immediate impairments in function. Impairments in function occur only when the disease has progressed to interference with the delivery of adequate amounts of blood to the organ or tissues involved. Many years may elapse between the first appearance of the disease and its progression to the point where an adequate blood flow can no longer be maintained.

In young animals, arteries display a high degree of elasticity which is associated with the collagen and elastin contained in their walls. With aging, arteries become thicker and less elastic. The gradual loss of elasticity increases the resistance offered to the flow of blood through the vessel so that a higher pressure must be maintained by the heart to keep the same amount of blood flowing.

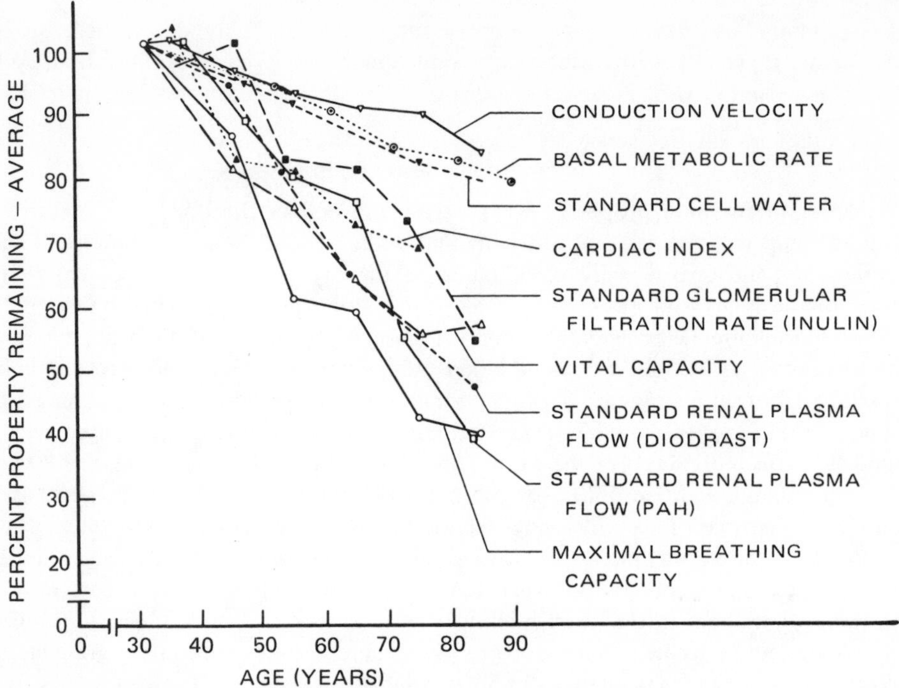


**Fig. 5**—A graph compares by age the functioning in a group of males of various vital processes of the body—nervous system, cell activity, heartbeat, kidney function and respiratory system. For each function, values are expressed as the percent of the mean value for subjects 25–35 years.

Average values for systolic and diastolic blood pressure obtained from measurements made on a large number of subjects tested in connection with the National Health Survey show a gradual increase with age (Table 4). This population undoubtedly included subjects with undiagnosed hypertension, obesity, and other conditions which increase blood pressure. In contrast, studies on private patients who were judged by their physicians as free from hypertension and were not obese showed practically no rise in systolic blood pressure in men aged 60 years and above (average 130 mm Hg). In the absence of disease, blood pressure does not increase significantly with age.

**TABLE 4**
**MEAN BLOOD PRESSURE IN ADULTS BY AGE AND SEX**

| | Men | | Women | |
|---|---|---|---|---|
| **Age** | **Systolic mm.** | **Diastolic mm.** | **Systolic mm.** | **Diastolic mm.** |
| 18–24 years | 121.7 | 71.6 | 111.8 | 69.4 |
| 25–34 years | 124.7 | 76.4 | 115.6 | 72.9 |
| 35–44 years | 128.6 | 80.7 | 122.8 | 78.0 |
| 45–54 years | 133.8 | 83.2 | 133.8 | 82.0 |
| 55–64 years | 140.3 | 83.1 | 146.6 | 84.9 |
| 65–74 years | 148.0 | 81.0 | 160.2 | 83.7 |
| 75–79 years | 154.3 | 79.4 | 156.6 | 79.3 |

Source: U. S. Public Health Service.

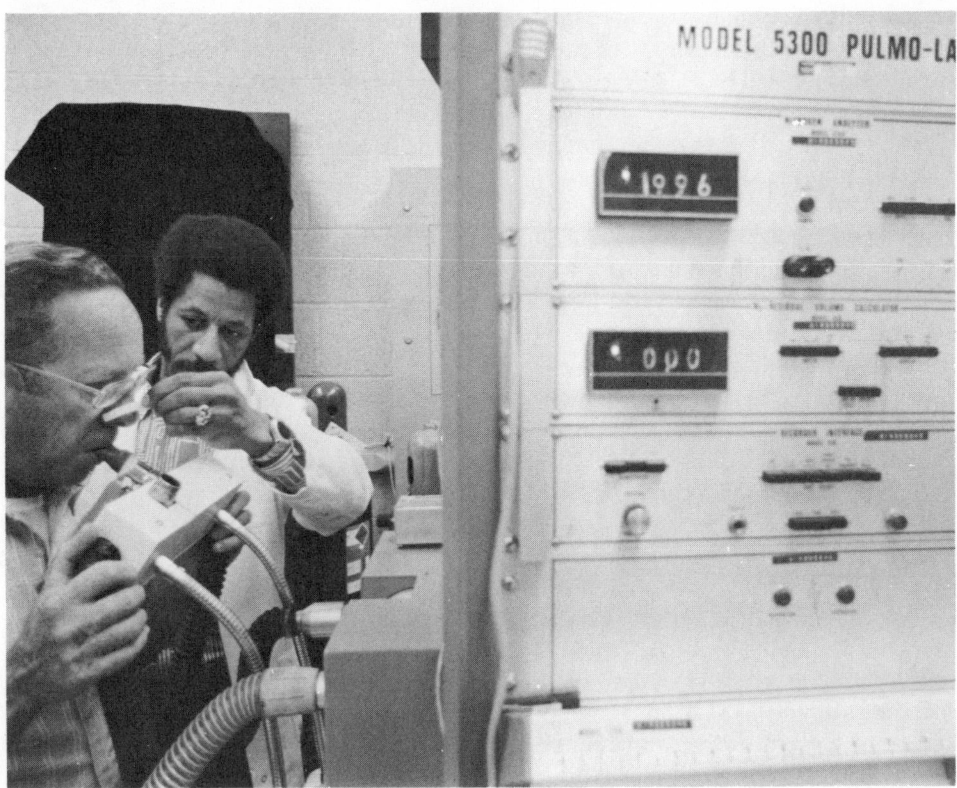


No part of the body escapes the aging process. The Pulmo-Lab measures the changes in lung function that occur with age. The man is one of more than 600 community volunteers taking part in long-term studies of aging at the Gerontology Research Center in Baltimore.

On the average, obese people have higher blood pressures than those of normal body weight. Since the incidence of obesity increases with age at least up to the age of 55–60, this factor may contribute to the increase in blood pressure with age observed in a general population.

### KIDNEY FUNCTION

Blood flow to the kidney diminishes with age. Part of the reduction is due to the fall in cardiac output, but there is, in addition, a physiological constriction of the blood vessels in the kidney which further restricts blood flow through the kidney.

A gradual reduction occurs with age in the ability of the kidney to produce urine. The amount of filtrate formed by the kidney per minute is reduced and the urine excreted is more dilute in the old than in the young. Consequently, the volume of urine excreted each 24 hours may be increased in the aged. However, the reductions in kidney function do not seriously impair excretion, since waste products removed by the kidney do not accumulate in the blood stream of normal elderly people.

### LUNG FUNCTION

Vital capacity, or the total amount of air that can be expelled from the lungs after a maximum inspiration, diminishes with age as does the total volume of air that is contained in the lungs. In contrast, the amount of air that cannot be voluntarily expelled from the lungs increases. These changes in respiratory mechanics are primarily a reflection of increased stiffness of the bony cage of the chest and the decreased strength of the muscles that move the chest during respiration.

The transfer of oxygen and carbon dioxide between the air in the lungs and the blood is influenced by the amount of blood flowing through the lungs as well as by the amount of air moved in and out. Although the amount of blood flowing through the lungs is reduced in the elderly, it is only under conditions of strenuous exercise that the older subject suffers from a lack of oxygen, that is, under conditions where very large amounts of oxygen are needed. There is no evidence that elderly people suffer from a chronic lack of oxygen.

Emphysema, the abnormal distension of the lungs with air, is a lung disease reaching its highest incidence between the ages of 45 and 65. In the United States the death rate from emphysema increased by almost 400 percent between 1950 and 1960. Although the exact causes of the disease are still unknown, the presence of noxious or toxic agents in the air may be a contributing factor. Many studies have shown that the incidence of emphysema and bronchitis is higher among smokers than non-smokers. Among British physicians death rates from bronchitis were six times higher in those smoking 25 cigarettes a day than in non-smokers.

Tests of lung function are significantly poorer in cigarette smokers than in non-smokers. Actually, cigarette smokers show values from any tests of lung function which are characteristic of non-smokers who are approximately 10 years older. In serial measurements made over a period of 10 years in the same person it was possible to compare pre- and post-smoking values for lung function tests made in people who stopped smoking. Cigarette smokers who stopped smoking improved with respect to lung function to the level attained by non-smokers within a period of 12–18 months after they had stopped. Even in habitual smokers improvements in lung function can be expected if the person drops this habit.

### SKELETAL SYSTEM

The bones of the body gradually lose calcium with advancing age. As a result they become more fragile and are more likely to break, even with minor falls. Healing of fractures is also slower in the old than in the young. However, recent advances in orthopedic surgery have made possible replacement of parts of the broken bone or joint with a new structure or introduction of a metallic peg to hold broken parts together. Osteoporosis, a disease characterized by the loss of calcium and minerals from bones, also increases with age. It occurs more frequently in women after menopause than in men and is especially evident in the spinal column.

### NERVOUS SYSTEM

Measurable physiological changes in the nervous system with age are relatively small. For example, the speed of conduction of nerve impulses falls by only about 10 percent over the age span of 30 to 80 years. This decrease is much too small to account for the longer reaction times observed in the elderly. This slowing of responses is most likely associated with the transmission of nerve impulses within the brain. There is also a loss of neurones (nerve cells) in the brain. However, the total number of nerve cells in the brain is so large that the losses are probably of little consequence with respect to mental functions. Since the physiological basis of memory

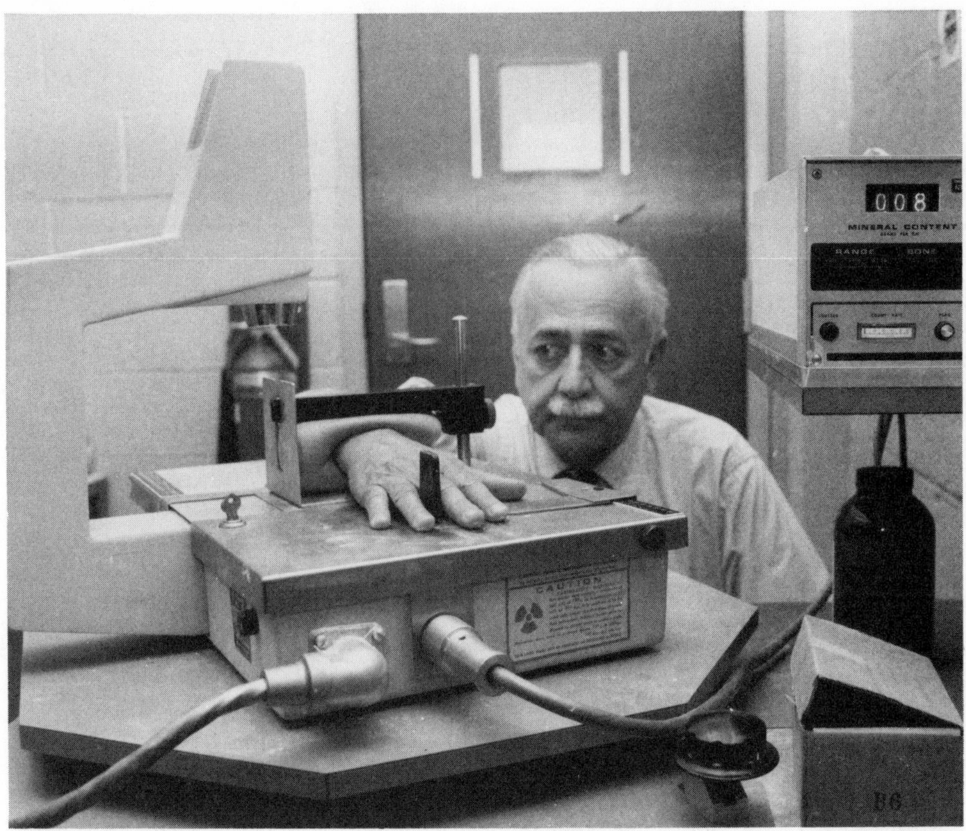


A gradual diminishing of calcium and minerals makes the bones of the elderly more brittle and thus easier to break and slower to heal. Science is working to understand the process in order to develop ways of controlling it. In a test to measure the rate of bone loss, a narrow beam is scanning the man's forearm to analzye the mineral content and width of the bones. The data are processed through a computer which reads out an index of density on the machine at right.

is still unknown, it cannot be assumed that the loss of memory often observed in elderly people is caused by the loss of neurones from the brain.

Neurones are extremely sensitive to oxygen deficiency. Consequently, any changes in the brain which interfere with its blood supply and thus reduce delivery of oxygen may have significant effects on brain functions. Although the total blood flow to the brain shows only a small decrease with advancing age, flow may be substantially reduced in small localized areas which may account for some of the age decrements in mental functions.

Undoubtedly there are functional changes in the brain and nervous system which are still not measurable and account for the slowing of responses and the memory defects which are often seen in the elderly. Even small changes in the transmission of impulses within the brain could markedly alter intellectual functions, but until more is known about how the brain works, relationships between brain function and behavior will remain obscure. It is apparent that because of the slow course of aging and the adaptability of the nervous system, adequate function is maintained in many individuals to advanced ages.

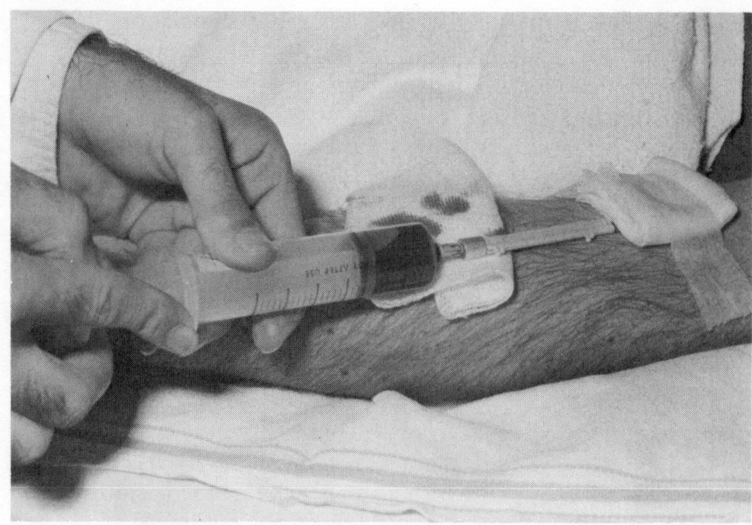

A blood sample is taken from the arm of a man undergoing a two-hour procedure testing his body's use of sugar. At the start of the test, a sugar solution is swallowed or injected into a vein. He has undergone this test for many years in a study to learn how sugar metabolism changes with age.

ENDOCRINE SYSTEM

Because of the importance of hormones in regulating many physiological functions, impairments in the endocrine glands have been traditionally regarded as important determinants of aging.

The hormone secreted by the thyroid gland (thyroxine) regulates the rate of chemical reactions in all cells of the body. When thyroxine secretion is reduced, the rate of chemical reactions and the uptake of oxygen is reduced. The basal metabolic rate is a measurement which indicates the total amount of oxygen being taken up by all of the cells of the body. Since basal metabolism decreases with age, it seems reasonable to ascribe aging to a reduction in the production of thyroxine. However, this is not the case. Experimental studies have shown that the reduction in basal metabolism is, for the most part, a reflection of the loss of tissue and cells in the aged. The oxygen uptake of the cells remaining in the body does not diminish with age. At the cellular level there is no evidence for a slowing of metabolism in old people. Although the rate of production of thyroxine diminishes with age, this is not due to impairment in the ability of the thyroid gland to produce thyroxine, since thyroxine production can be increased as much in the old as in the young when thyroid stimulating hormone is administered experimentally. With advancing age, tissues of the body use less thyroxine. With the reduced requirement, the thyroid gland simply produces less of the hormone.

Since aging is associated with reduced ability to adjust to stresses and since the adrenal cortex plays a role in many of these adjustments, numerous attempts have been made to assess age changes in the adrenal gland. Although there is a reduction in the urinary excretion of the breakdown products of adrenal cortical hormones, the ability of the gland to produce hormones when stimulated by the experimental administration of the pituitary hormone that regulates the activity of the adrenal cortex indicates that the response is as good in the old as in the young. Aging does not seem to produce any significant impairment in the adrenal gland.

The pituitary gland is often referred to as the master gland of the body, since it produces a number of hormones that regulate the activity of other endocrine glands, such as the adrenal, thyroid, ovary and testis. Therefore, it is possible that the age reduction in the function of these glands is due to the lack of proper stimulation from the pituitary gland. Unfortunately, analytical methods for determining the very small amounts of these regulating hormones that are present in the blood have been developed only recently and systematic studies of age differences in blood levels of these regulatory hormones have not been reported, so that the question is still unanswered.

With advancing age there is significant reduction in the rate of removal of excess sugar from the blood. In young people this serves as a diagnostic criterion for the presence of diabetes, a disease which is due to inadequate production of insulin by the pancreas. At present it is not known whether this reduction in glucose tolerance in older people represents the early stages of diabetes or whether it is a normal age change. It does appear in aged individuals who do not show any clinical symptoms of diabetes. Furthermore, it has been shown that, unlike the diabetic, elderly subjects can, with additional stimulation, release more insulin. In young persons, the pancreas releases more insulin in response to even a slight rise in blood sugar levels than occurs in the elderly. In the elderly, the sensitivity of the pancreas is reduced so that a higher level of blood sugar is required to stimulate it to action. With maximum stimulation the pancreas of the aged can produce as much insulin as the pancreas of the young. The age deficit in the pancreas lies not in its ability to produce or release insulin, but in its reduced sensitivity to the stimulus—a rise in blood sugar level.

Youthful virility in males has long been regarded as a behavioral characteristic that is dependent on the secretion of male sex hormones. Attempts to rejuvenate middle-aged and elderly males by the injection of extracts of testicular tissue or the transplantation of sex glands from young males, goats, and monkeys reflected this belief. As stated before, none of these procedures were successful in providing lasting benefits and have now been abandoned by responsible physicians.

Numerous studies have shown that the excretion of male sex hormones and their metabolic products falls gradually with advancing age.

Blood levels of testosterone in men increase considerably from adolescence to early adulthood and remain relatively stable up to the age of 50 years. After this age there is a gradual fall so that by age 80–90 mean levels are only about 40 percent of the values found before age 50. There is no evidence that testosterone secretion drops rapidly after a given age which would be comparable to the rapid fall in female sex hormone production in women which occurs at the menopause. Individual differences in blood levels of testosterone are great. Some 80-year-olds have blood levels of testosterone which exceed the mean values found in 20-year-olds. No studies are as yet available which can specify the relationships between sexual functioning, age, and blood levels of testosterone in specific individuals.

### SEXUAL ACTIVITY OF THE AGED

Although sexual interest, drive, and vigor in the adult male decline with advancing age, these behavioral characteristics cannot be ascribed entirely to decreasing secretion of testosterone. In humans, sexual behavior is determined more by social and cultural factors than by physiological states. Recent studies, based on interview reports and questionnaires, indicate that sexual activity continued to play an important role in the lives of many elderly people and that the primary factors determining continued sexual activity were (1) the level of sexual functioning in younger years,

(2) the enjoyment derived at younger ages, (3) the availability of a sexual partner, (4) continuity of sexual activity, and (5) general health status. In one study, one-fifth of the men in their 80's and 90's reported continued sexual activity. The current social taboo against sexual activity after age 60 plays an important role in sexual behavior in the elderly. In the eyes of society, what is regarded as virility at 25 becomes lechery at 65. With changing attitudes toward sex, patterns of sexual activity among older people may change remarkably.

### IMPOTENCE

Clinical reports indicate that the incidence of impotence increases with age. However, no comprehensive data are available to permit valid estimates of its prevalence in the population. Clinical studies indicate that the condition is more apt to be based on psychological problems than on physiological deficits. Appropriate counseling and psychotherapy are regarded as more appropriate forms of treatment than the administration of testosterone. There is no evidence that prostatectomy induces impotence. In one study of 68 potent men subjected to prostatectomy 84 percent retained potency after the operation.

### HORMONES AND THE MENOPAUSE

In women, blood levels of female sex hormones produced by the ovary fall markedly at the menopause. This drop is a reflection of the physiological changes in the ovary associated with the cessation of the production and release of ova. Although it is assumed that this is due to exhaustion of the supply of cells (oocytes) which produce ova, details of the mechanisms involved are still unknown. When ovulation ceases and the amount of female sex hormones released is reduced, menstruation stops. Some women experience other physiological disturbances, such as headaches, dizziness and hot flashes, but the physiological mechanisms for these phenomena are still unknown.

There is still considerable controversy about the desirability of treating post-menopausal women with periodic injections of female sex hormones. Some physicians believe that this therapy can improve the overall well-being of women by replacing the female sex hormones which have been greatly reduced at the menopause. However, other physicians argue that the effects are minimal and the hazards are great, since it has been well established that, at least in animals, the steroid hormones, including the female sex hormone, can induce cancer.

Little information is available on sexual behavior in older women. A classic study on sexual behavior in women included data on only 56 women over the age of 60, but the authors concluded that there was "little evidence of aging of sexual capacity in females until late in life." More recent studies indicate that, although sexual interest is less in women than in men, it does not disappear. In fact, some women reported an increase in interest after the menopause which continued into the 60's and 70's. Continuation of sexual activity in later life depended in large measure on the level of interest and degree of satisfaction derived during early and middle life. A primary requirement for maintenance of sexual capacity and effective sexual performance is the opportunity for regular sexual expression. In view of the high incidence of widowhood among aging females, their opportunities for sexual expression become increasingly restricted. In general, it seems that there are no physiological limits to female sexuality that are imposed by advancing years. The primary limits are related to social standards and personality characteristics.

### IMMUNE SYSTEM

The immune system protects the body against disease. The system consists of the lymph nodes, spleen, thymus, tonsils, and Peyer's patches of the bowel, as well as the bone marrow. In general, the system serves to inactivate, localize, or destroy foreign substances which gain entry into the body, whether these substances are toxic chemicals, living microorganisms such as bacteria or viruses, or products of living organisms such as toxins or enzymes. The general mechanism of the immune response is the production of antibodies which destroy a specific foreign substance and are formed by sensitized cells (lymphocytes) or other plasma cells which are derived from lymphocytes. The process involves at least two important stages: a recognition that a chemical, an organism, or cell is a foreign substance, i.e., not a normal part of the individual; and the production of an appropriate antibody or cell which will neutralize the foreign substance. With increasing age the ability to form antibodies is diminished, the rate of production is slowed, and the total amount of the antibody produced is reduced. This finding can explain in part the increased susceptibility of older people to a variety of infectious diseases.

It is also possible that the process whereby the immune system recognizes a foreign substance is impaired so that the process of antibody formation is not initiated. It is now believed by some that the increased incidence of cancer in older people may be due to the failure of the immune system to recognize aberrant cancerous cells in the body and destroy them. The result is that these aberrant cells divide and reproduce in uncontrolled fashion resulting in the development of cancer. Although this conception has not been proved, it is an attractive hypothesis and considerable research is in progress to test it.

Under normal circumstances, the body possesses a built-in mechanism which prevents it from developing antibodies against its own cells or tissues. For example, a rabbit will readily respond to the injection of an extract of rat kidney with a production of antibodies directed against rat kidney. It will even develop antibodies to cells or tissues taken from another rabbit. In spite of this, the rabbit does not normally make antibodies against its own kidneys. However, under certain circumstances these protective mechanisms break down and an animal may produce antibodies which act upon its own tissues and cells. When this happens a so-called autoimmune disease develops. A number of such diseases have been identified. Certain kinds of hemolytic anemias are the consequence of antibody mediated cytotoxic reactions directed against the subject's own red blood cells.

This mechanism of autoimmunity has been proposed as the cause of cell death and of aging. Although still unproven, it is a provocative hypothesis and one which can be tested experimentally. Furthermore, if aging turns out to be related to autoimmunity, the rapidly advancing knowledge about immunity may lead to procedures which can retard the effects of aging.

## PATTERNS OF AGING

Aging does not influence all organ systems to the same extent. Some physiological characteristics remain unchanged even into the 80's and 90's. For example, fasting

**TABLE 5**
**MEAN SERUM CHOLESTEROL LEVELS**

| Age | Male | | Female | |
|---|---|---|---|---|
| | Mean | Std Dev. | Mean | Std Dev. |
| 18–24 years | 178.1 | 47.9 | 184.7 | 47.9 |
| 25–34 years | 205.9 | 44.6 | 197.9 | 41.9 |
| 35–44 years | 226.8 | 49.4 | 213.6 | 45.3 |
| 45–54 years | 230.5 | 45.6 | 236.8 | 50.0 |
| 55–64 years | 232.8 | 49.0 | 262.3 | 63.0 |
| 65–74 years | 229.5 | 47.3 | 265.7 | 58.8 |
| 75–79 years | 224.5 | 48.7 | 245.3 | 65.7 |

*(mg/100 ml)
Source: *National Health Survey*. U. S. Department of Health, Education, and Welfare, National Center for Health Statistics.

blood sugar levels, the acidity of the blood, blood protein, and the total blood volume do not change significantly between the ages of 30 and 80. Close regulation of these characteristics of the blood is essential in maintaining the proper internal environment for functioning cells. The body has available a number of mechanisms to regulate these characteristics and to maintain them within fairly close limits under resting conditions even in old people. When displacements in blood sugar level, acidity, etc. do occur as a result of physiological stresses such as disease, exercise, food ingestion, and the like, old people require more time to readjust to basal or resting levels than do the young.

### CHOLESTEROL LEVELS

Another pattern of aging shows a period of increasing values throughout middle life with decrements only after middle age. An example of this pattern is the level of cholesterol in the blood. At age 20 average values are about 178 mg percent in men and 185 mg percent in women. Values for men rise progressively and reach a maximum of about 232 mg percent at age 55 to 60 after which there is a fall to about 224 mg percent at age 75 (Table 5).

Although the average values decline after age 60, it cannot be assumed that blood cholesterol levels fall in an individual as he ages. This is because it is possible that individuals with high values die at a greater rate than individuals with low values so that they no longer are included in the averages computed for higher age groups. In other words, age changes in an individual can be determined only by making repeated measurements on the same subject as he ages. Such a longitudinal study has been in progress at the Gerontology Research Center, Baltimore, since 1959. This study involves some 650 men aged 20 to 96 who have been tested every 18 months. The subjects are all normal individuals living in the community who come to the GRC for two and a half days of testing every 18 months. An extensive battery of clinical, physiological, biochemical, and psychological tests are administered to each subject. The study is still in progress, but preliminary analyses show that individual subjects, aged 60 and over, show a gradual lowering of blood cholesterol levels in contrast to subjects aged 20 to 60, who show rising levels.

Most physiological functions show a gradual decrement that extends over the entire life span. Because of the wide range in measurements found in individuals at each age decade, the average trend with age can be represented as a straight line.

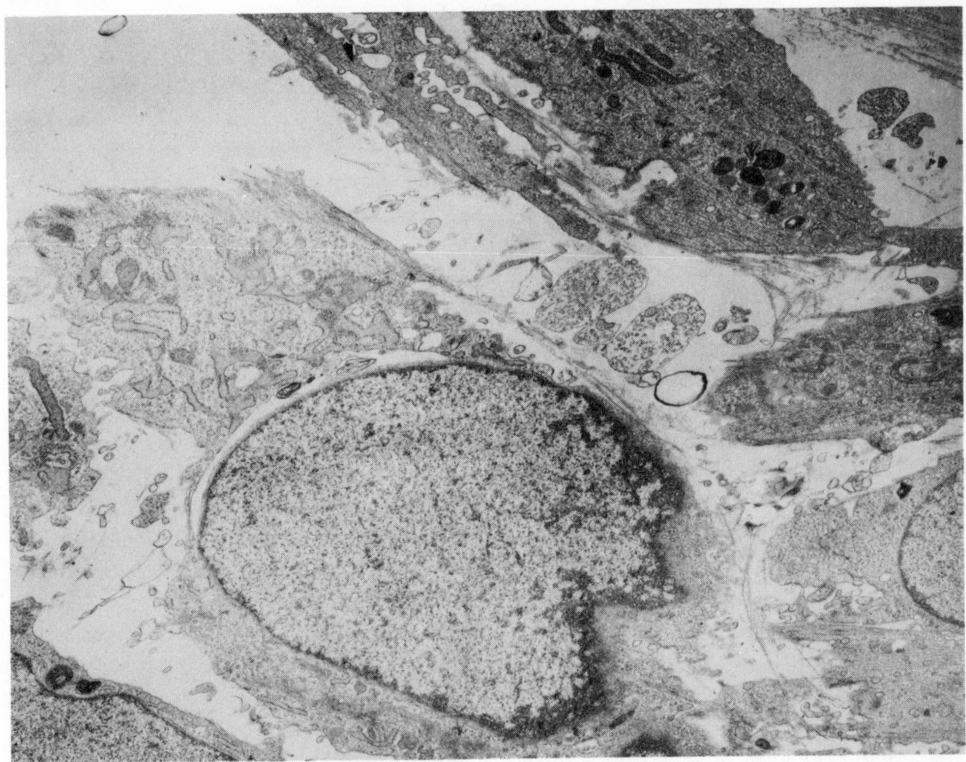

Death of irreplaceable cells in certain body organ tissues is one of the reasons some functions decrease with age, and the answer to why individual cells die is under intense study by scientists. Cell study has been greatly advanced by technological developments such as electron microscopy, which allows far greater magnification than ordinary microscopes. This is a transmission electron micrograph of IMR-90 cells—a cell line specially cultured for aging research.

Figure 5 compares the average age trends for a number of physiological tests. In this figure, the average value for 30-year-olds is taken as 100 percent. Subsequent values up to age 85 are shown as the percent decrement for each variable. The decrements between age 30 and 85 vary widely for different physiological functions. For example, the decrement in the speed of conduction of a nerve impulse falls by only 10 percent over the age span of 30 to 85 years while cardiac output falls 40 percent, kidney function 50 percent, and maximum breathing capacity 60 percent over the same age range. These results show that aging is not a uniform process that affects all organ systems at the same rate.

## ROLE OF CELL LOSS IN AGING

One of the causes for these age decrements is that in some organs individual cells or functioning units simply die and drop out. In organs such as the heart, muscle, and the nervous system, cells, once lost, cannot be replaced. Consequently, these losses are cumulative and result in a loss of reserve capacities in that organ. It should, however, be pointed out that all the organs of the body have a great many more cells and functioning units than are required for normal existence. For example, if one kidney is surgically removed the remaining kidney contains a sufficient number of functioning units to maintain the individual under normal circumstances. There is, furthermore, a hypertrophy of the cells in the remaining kidney so that within a month or so normal function has been restored. Similarily, some two-thirds of the liver can be removed and regeneration will occur, even in old animals. The only effect of age is that slightly more time may be required for regeneration in the old than in the young animal. Thus these losses, while they may reduce reserve capacities, are not large enough to threaten normal existence. At present, the cause of death of individual cells within a tissue is not known, but this represents an intensive area of research that is being pursued by investigators in gerontology.

## ROLE OF CONTROL MECHANISMS

Performances which require the integrated activity of a number of organ systems show greater age decrements than do the performances of a single organ system. For example, performance of physical exercise requires the integrated activity of the heart, blood vessels, lungs, muscles, and nervous system. Experiments have shown that the maximum effects of aging appear in the rate at which exercise can be performed. The age decrement in the performance of a cranking operation which requires coordinated movements of the muscles of the arms or legs falls at a greater rate than does the strength of the individual muscles required to perform the work. Maximum breathing capacity, which requires coordinated movement to voluntarily increase the rate of breathing, falls more with age than the vital capacity, which requires only a single maximum expiration. These experiments and others lead to the conclusion that aging is the result of impairment in physiological control mechanisms.

## ADAPTATION TO STRESS

One outstanding characteristic of aging is a reduction in the ability to adjust to stressful situations. Physiologically, this characteristic appears as an increase in the time required by the older person to adjust to a stress. With exercise there is an increase in respiration, blood pressure, and heart rate which disappears with the cessation of the exercise. With increasing age the time required for the blood pressure, heart rate, and breathing to return to normal levels after exercise is greater in the old than in the young. When sugar is ingested the blood sugar level rises to a peak in about two hours and then returns to normal values after an additional hour. With increasing age the time required for the blood sugar to reach its resting levels is significantly increased. This reduction in speed of response even appears at a cellular level. For example, the rate at which some enzymes can be produced by the liver diminishes with advancing age. Wound healing progresses effectively in the aged but at a slower rate than in the young.

One of the most striking characteristics of aging is that more time is required to carry out many functions. In many instances, older individuals can achieve the same final performance as the middle-aged except that it takes them longer.

The slowing of responses in the elderly is also present in behavioral characteristics. Reaction times are longer in the old than in the young and the age differences are greater for choice reaction times (where the subject is presented with a number of stimuli but is instructed to respond to only one of them) than in simple reaction times (where only one stimulus is presented to which the subject must respond as quickly as he can). Learning is slower in the elderly and they have greater difficulty in dealing with situations where a number of stimuli must be identified and dealt with quickly, as for example, in dealing with multiple road signs while driving a car on a modern superhighway.

## BIOLOGICAL THEORIES OF AGING

Over the years many theories about the cause of aging have been proposed. Many of these theories attribute senescence to changes in specific organs or tissues, such as heart and blood vessels, nerve cells, endocrine glands, and so forth. The general assumption has been that cells and organs simply wear out as do machines. This basic assumption that animals are like machines is not in accord with biological facts, since all organisms have many built-in repair mechanisms which provide continuous replacement of enzymes and even cells in some organs, such as the skin, liver, and the digestive tract. At the present time there is no single theory that can explain all of the facts known about aging. However, with the advances made in molecular biology there are now some hypotheses about aging that seem reasonable and can be tested with laboratory experiments.

### GENETIC THEORY

One theory of aging assumes that the life span of a cell or organism is determined by its genes which contain a program that sets its life span just as certain genes determine eye color. The wide range of life spans among different animal species is clear evidence that some genetic program exists. Some insects have a total life span as short as one day. Rats and mice live two to three years, dogs twelve to fifteen, and humans about 70 years. Even within a species genetic differences may play a role. In both mice and fruit flies selective breeding has made it possible to produce separate strains with relatively long and short life spans. It has been shown even in humans that individuals with parents and grandparents who have lived to the age of 70 will, on the average, live two to three years longer than individuals whose parents died before the age of 60.

### ERROR HYPOTHESIS

According to modern biological theory, the double helix of the DNA molecule located in the nucleus of the cell contains all of the information that is necessary for the assembly of the specific proteins from the constituent amino acids. This information resides in the DNA molecule in a coded form and depends on the order in which four primary nucleotides are attached to the spiral chains of the DNA molecule. The actual assembly of the appropriate amino acids to form specific proteins or enzymes is assumed to occur elsewhere in the cell, namely, on the ribosomes. In order to do this, information from the DNA must be transferred to an appropriate location on the ribosome. This transfer occurs by assembly of RNA molecules at a specific point on the DNA molecule, which then migrate to the ribosomes where the protein molecules are assembled.

This general theory of biology has been transferred to gerontology as the error hypothesis of cellular aging. According to this hypothesis, aging and death of a cell result from errors which may occur in any of the many steps in this sequence of information transfer. These errors may result in the formation of protein molecules which have small deviations in their structure so that they are unable to participate in chemical reactions which are essential for life of the cell. A wide variety of RNAs are formed in each cell depending on the protein or enzyme to be producd. Slight errors in the final protein could accumulate in the cell and eventually cause its death. Although some investigators claim to have observed differences in RNAs that have been isolated from old and young tissues, the detection of atypical proteins, that is, those with errors, has been much more difficult. The error hypothesis is, however, a viable one which makes predictions about aging and which can be tested experimentally.

### SOMATIC MUTATION

As cells grow and divide a small proportion of them undergo mutation, that is, they become different, with a change in their genetic structure that is then reproduced when they again divide. The somatic mutation hypothesis assumes that these atypical cells are unable to carry out the normal function of the cell, so that as they accumulate with age, the function of the organ deteriorates and ultimately the animal dies. Evidence for this hypothesis is based primarily on the life-shortening effects of exposure to radiation. Exposure to radiation greatly accelerates the rate of mutation in most cell populations. Furthermore, it has been shown repeatedly that exposure to a non-lethal dose of radiation will shorten the life span in experimental animals as well as in humans. Although this hypothesis has enjoyed some popularity in the past, more detailed mathematical analysis has shown that the rate of mutation in somatic cells is probably not high enough to account for observed changes with age. Furthermore, the somatic mutation hypothesis is focused primarily on dividing cells (a mutation can only occur when a cell divides) whereas aging is a process which involves changes with time in cells which do not divide. Although the hypothesis may account for the life-shortening effects of exposure to radiation, it does not seem to explain cellular aging.

### DEPRIVATION AND ACCUMULATION HYPOTHESES

Other theories of aging focus attention on factors that can influence the expression of the genetically determined program. One of these is the wear and tear theory discussed previously. Although aging may reduce the effectiveness of cellular repair mechanisms in the elderly, it is doubtful whether the concept of "wearing out" is applicable to a living system.

It has also been assumed that aging results from a gradual reduction in the delivery of oxygen and nutrients to the cells of the body. This may occur where parts of the circulation become blocked and specific areas of a tissue or organ fail to receive an adequate supply of blood. However, under these conditions a substantial group of cells die. These effects are due to disease processes affecting blood vessels and are quite different from the cell loss associated with aging, where the lost cells are more or less randomly distributed in an organ or tissue. Studies on age changes in blood oxygen levels or blood concentrations of various nutrients fail to show a progressive fall, so that there is no evidence to support the deprivation theories of cellular aging.

A corollary to the wear and tear theory is the presumption that waste products accumulate within cells and interfere with their function and ultimately result in death.

The accumulation of highly insoluble particles known as age pigments has been observed in muscle cells in the heart and nerve cells of both human beings and other animals. However, it has not been demonstrated that the presence of these particles interferes with cellular function.

### CROSS-LINKING THEORY

With the passage of time many macromolecules of biological importance develop cross-linkages or bonds either between component parts of the same molecule or between different molecules. The formation of these cross-links alters the physical and chemical properties of many large molecules so they no longer function the same way as before. Since these cross-links are very stable and accumulate with the passage of time, one theory holds with this as a primary cause of aging. Most of the experimental evidence supporting this theory has been derived through studies on connective tissue and collagen. From these observed facts with respect to collagen it has been assumed that similar changes occur in intracellular proteins as well. These cross-links could alter the structure and shape of the enzyme molecules in a cell so they are no longer able to carry out their functions. The formation of cross-links in intracellular proteins has not yet been demonstrated. However, the theory is a viable one which may well explain molecular changes which form the basis for known changes in the characteristics of the structural proteins at least. The theory leads to an experimental approach to discover methods whereby cross-links, once formed, may be broken down and, perhaps more importantly, the methods which would reduce their rate of formation in the animal.

## PROSPECTS FOR INCREASING LONGEVITY

It is highly improbable that the human life span can be doubled, that is, extended to 140–150 years, within the foreseeable future. This is because any large increase in life span will probably require a change in the basic genetic characteristics of individuals. Although research in basic biology ultimately may lead to methods for altering genetic characteristics, it is unlikely that such techniques can be applied to humans for a long time to come.

We can, however, expect bio-medical advances which will lead to prevention and control of many diseases which now limit life span. In addition, general improvement in socioeconomic living conditions throughout the world will continue to improve with a further reduction in mortality rates. These advances will result in the gradual increase in average age of death. We can also look for more and more people to approach their full genetically determined life span.

Old age itself is never the immediate cause of death. Rather, animals and humans die of many different diseases. The primary causes of death in rats are lung and kidney disease. This species does not spontaneously develop arteriosclerosis and heart disease. In contrast, the primary causes of death in humans are heart and blood vessel diseases followed by cancer. Since diseases represent the major cause of death, research leading to the prevention and improved treatment for a variety of diseases will have a major impact on length of life in the future. Before the discovery of insulin, diabetic patients lived only 5–6 years after developing the disease. The introduction of insulin and improved methods for the treatment of diabetes greatly increased the life span of these patients so that currently diabetics have an average life span only 10 years less than non-diabetics. It has been estimated that the elimination of heart and blood vessel diseases as causes of death would add around 8 years to the average life span. The elimination of cancer would add another 3 years. It is apparent, therefore, that the fruits of bio-medical research may add another 8–10 years of average life span within the next 25–30 years.

Claims are often made that certain treatments will minimize the effects of aging and significantly increase life span. For example, it is claimed that repeated injections of Gerovital (procaine) slow down the effects of aging. These claims stem largely from the Romanian literature, which is based entirely upon the reported improvement of patients receiving the therapy. No carefully controlled experiments have been reported. Furthermore, investigators in other countries, as well as in the United States, have been unable to demonstrate any effects of the drug when other factors are controlled.

The injection of suspensions of cells made from the organs of fetal sheep has also been publicized as a treatment for aging. A number of famous people reportedly were treated by Professor Niehans in his clinic in Switzerland. Actually, injection of fetal cells can now be obtained in a number of clinics in Europe. Here again, no carefully controlled experiments have been conducted and, since the treatment is potentially dangerous because of the immunological responses which the patient may develop,

Continuing research into the aging process in order to render meaningful assistance to older people includes the vital area of blood pressure. The man seen through the overhead mirror is learning to raise and lower his blood pressure through conditioning and feedback techniques. The equipment shown enables the scientist to monitor the subject's progress.

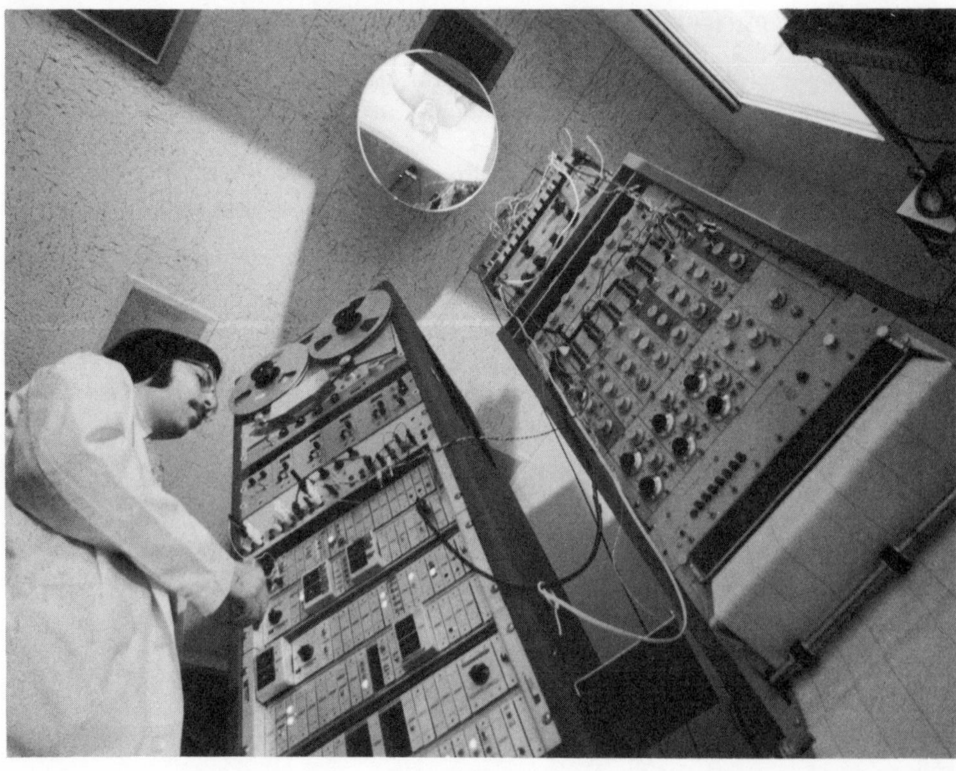

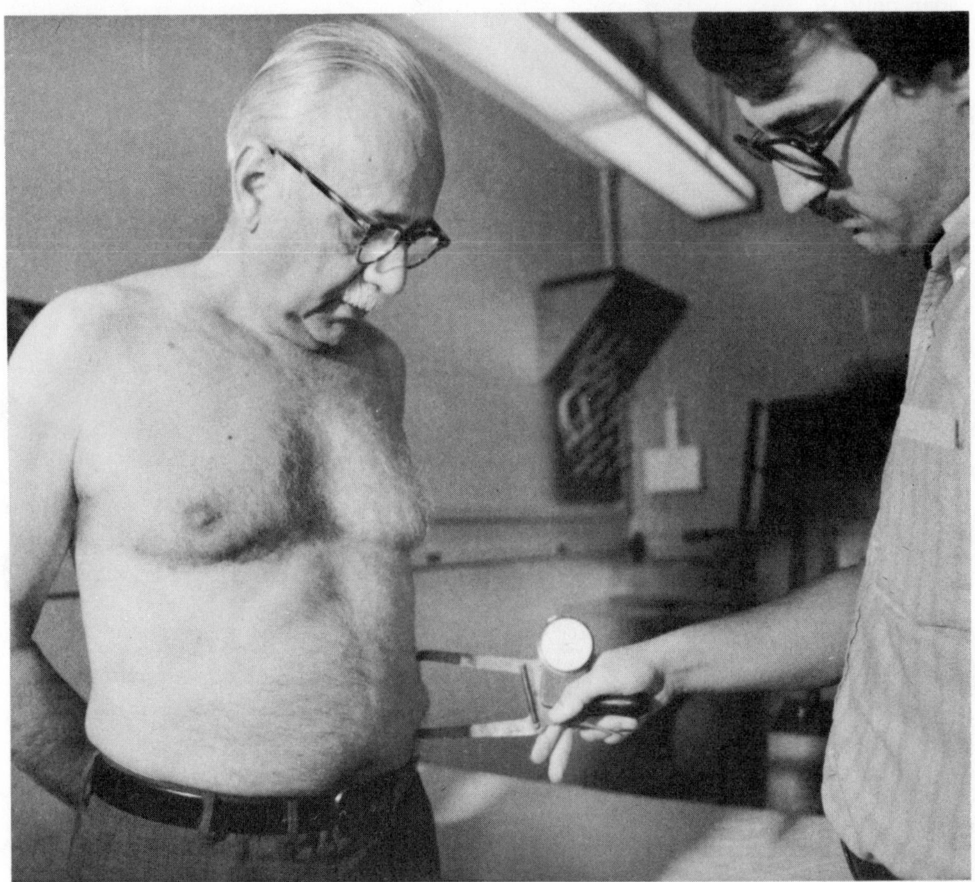

Because of the body's tendency to add fat as one grows older, the elderly are advised to beware of obesity and its problems. A participant in a long-term aging study, this man's body composition has been tested for nearly 20 years so that researchers can compare weight gain or fluctuation with physiological changes. Fat at his waistline is being measured with calipers, though it has been found that tape measurement of the waistline is a better indicator of fatness.

the treatment is not permitted in the United States. There is no solid evidence that either of these treatments can retard aging.

We have, however, gained knowledge which, if appropriately applied, can have an impact on health and vigor in the later years. It is now well known that obesity is associated with increased incidence of many diseases ranging from arthritis to hypertension, cardiovascular disease, and diabetes. On the average, individuals who are 25 percent overweight have a life expectancy of 3½ years less than subjects of normal weight. In markedly obese persons (60–65 percent overweight) life span may be reduced by as much as 15 years. Blood pressure is also significantly higher in subjects who are 20 percent or more overweight. High blood pressure also greatly increases the risk of developing heart disease. The elimination of obesity within a population would undoubtedly have a marked effect on health and life span.

Although there is little evidence of special dietary needs in the later years, it is clear that adequate nutrition, especially with respect to vitamins and trace elements, will have a major impact on health. Since caloric intake gradually diminishes over

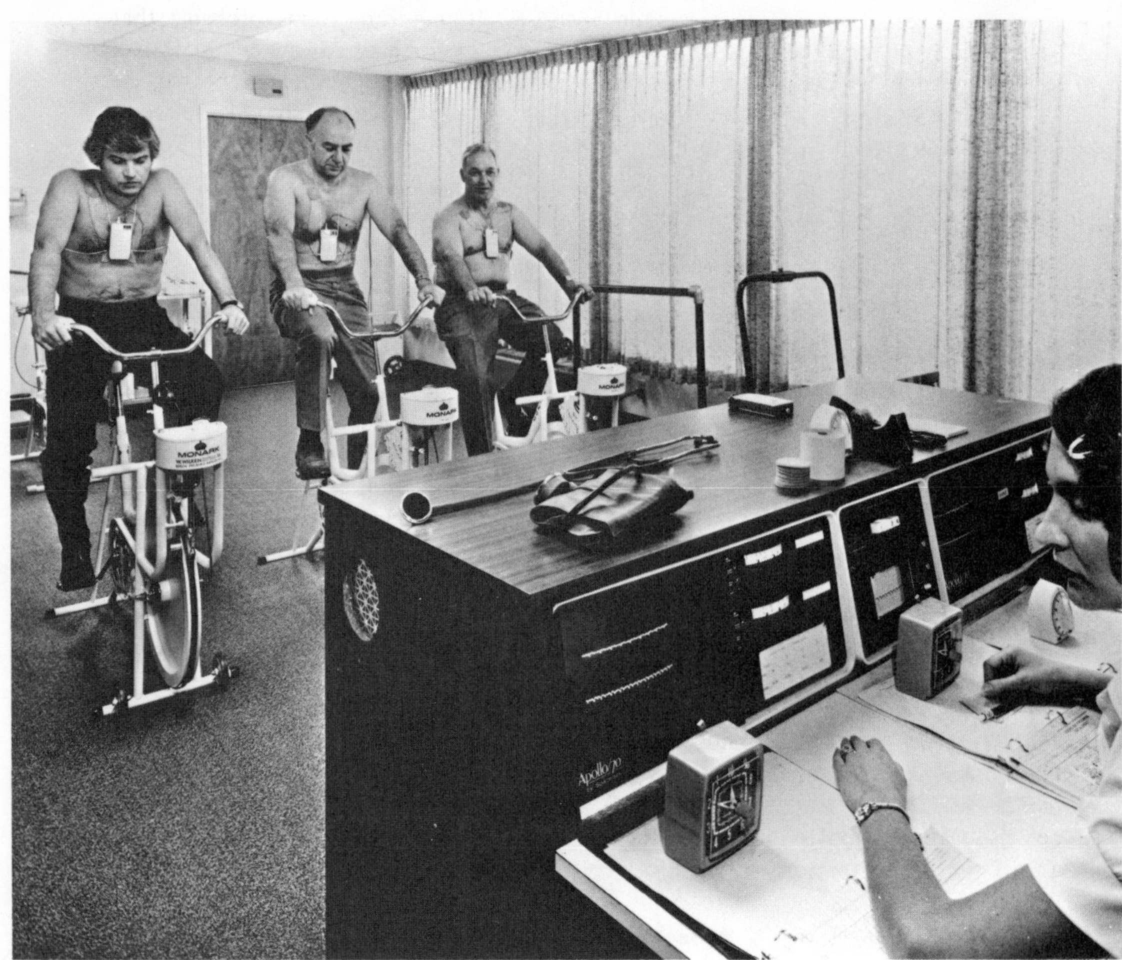


A bicycle stress test is being used to compare the heart rates of the middle-aged men with that of the young man at left. Sensors attached to their chests pick up the vital information, which is monitored by the technician at the console. Older people are being encouraged to develop regular habits of moderate exercise to stimulate blood flow and maintain muscular function.

a life span, the intake of vitamins and trace elements may become marginal in advanced old age simply because the quantity of food eaten is reduced. It is therefore possible that elderly subjects may benefit from vitamin supplements. The relationship between fat intake in the diet, blood cholesterol, and the development of atherosclerosis is not clearly defined. However, current evidence leads to the conclusion that intake of fat in the diet may well be reduced in the later years.

Although there is no evidence that those who participated in athletic activities during early life live any longer than non-participants, exercise is regarded by many as an effective device to minimize the effects of aging. At present there is no clear-cut experimental evidence to indicate that this is so. However, the known physiological effects of exercise in stimulating blood flow and maintaining muscular function gives some credence to this supposition. It has also been shown that physical fitness as measured by work output or maximum oxygen uptake can be improved in elderly people through training and systematic exercises. It therefore seems probable that participation in some form of physical activity or exercise is advantageous. It can certainly counteract the atrophy of disuse which appears in many elderly people.

Although we still do not know the basic causes of aging, research has already yielded results which can lead to improvements in the health status of elderly people and thus more effective living in the later years. This is the ultimate goal of gerontology (the scientific study of aging), namely, to improve the quality of life rather than merely its length.

**AGLYCEMIA,** the absence of sugar in the blood. Because sugar is vital to all cell functions, its complete absence results in death in minutes. The condition is extremely rare. Low blood sugar is referred to as *hypoglycemia. See also* **medigraph** HYPOGLYCEMIA.

**AGNOSIA,** the loss of the ability to recognize the impressions of any of the senses. Those with *acoustic agnosia* cannot recognize the significance of sounds. Those with *finger agnosia* cannot indicate their own or someone else's fingers. In *tactile agnosia,* the victim cannot remember the feel of objects. In *time agnosia,* a loss of the sense of the passage of time and the succession of events takes place. Victims of *visual agnosia* cannot recognize familiar objects by sight, and often they fail to remember even close relatives.

▶ Vision Impairment, *Refractive Errors and Visual Anomalies,* 2938.

**AGORAPHOBIA.** *See* PHOBIAS.

**AGRANULOCYTOSIS,** a serious condition, fortunately rare, in which the *white cells* of the blood are destroyed faster than they can be produced. This is the reverse of *leukemia* (in which the white cells are produced in such overabundance that they overwhelm the other components of the blood). The danger of agranulocytosis is that the destroyed white cells include *granulocytes* —the largest portion of which are *neutrophiles,* those cells that fight infection. The destruction of neutrophiles is called *neutropenia.*

Without these cells, defense against bacterial infection is lessened not only from the outside but even from organisms already present in the body. These bacteria, previously kept under control by the action of neutrophiles, now multiply at great speed and invade tissues. The result is the rapid development of infectious open sores at areas where bacteria are harbored: mouth, rectum, vagina, gut, and skin. Blood infections also occur. Chills, fever, and prostration result.

In most cases, agranulocytosis seems to be caused by various chemicals or drugs to which the patient has developed a sensitivity. Drugs known to cause the condition include *aminopyrine* (*pyramidon*), *phenylbutazone, promazine,* some *antithyroid agents,* a few *antibiotics,* several *antihistamines, barbiturates, gold compounds,* and drugs containing *arsenic.* Although the proportion of people who develop the agranulocytosis reaction to these drugs is small, drug manufacturers list the possibility; and the physicians who prescribe these drugs follow their patients carefully for signs of the reaction. All reactions should be reported to the doctor, especially after taking prescription drugs.

A far smaller number of agranulocytosis cases seem to be caused not by chemicals but by active infections. The condition has been reported in *virus*

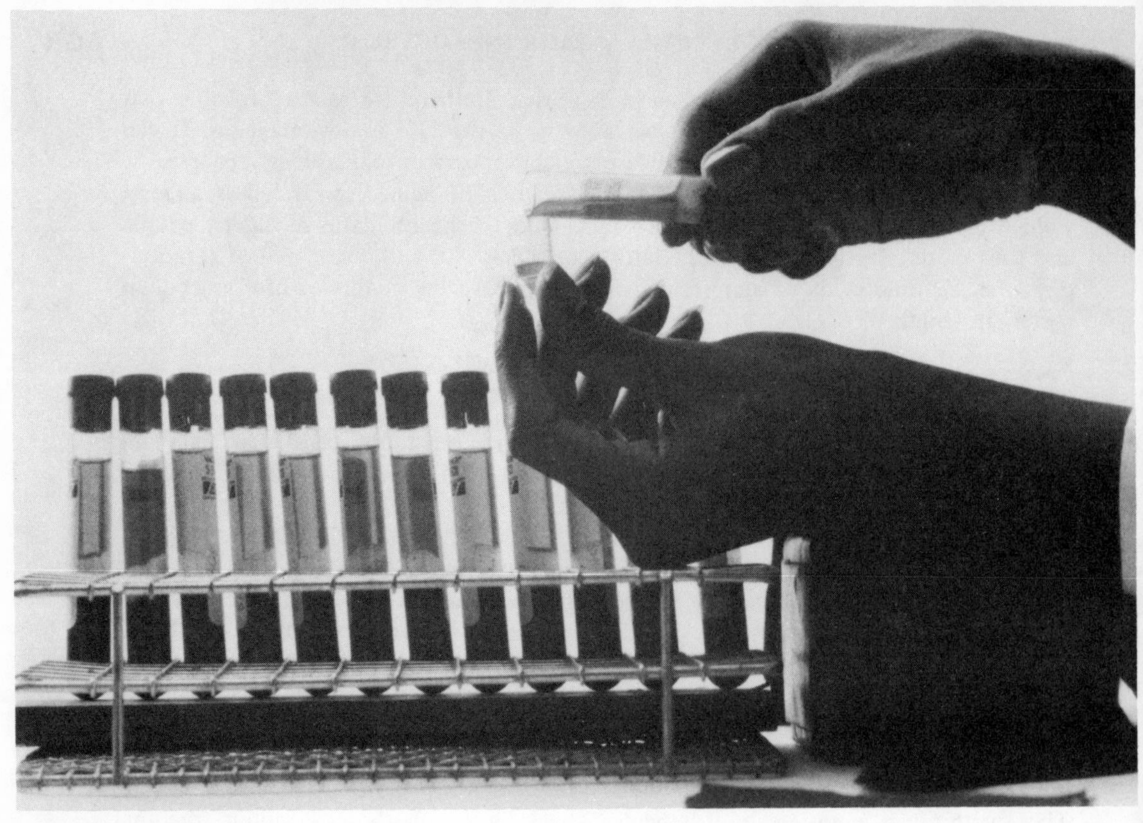

**Agranulocytosis**—A blood sample is being tested for this rare disease. Destruction of white blood cells leaves victims prey to open sores in mucuous membranes that harbor bacteria.

*pneumonia, infectious mononucleosis, Felty's syndrome,* and in *lupus erythematosus.*

Just how and where these chemical or infectious agents act on the granulocytes is not entirely known. While the destruction appears to take place in the small blood vessels, exhaustion and depletion of the special white cell-producing tissues develop in the bone marrow. Two or three times more women than men are affected.

Once, as many as 90 percent of those with the disease died of it. Such deaths are not common today, because modern antibiotics provide an effective weapon against it. The basis of the treatment is to identify what chemical or drug is responsible for the reaction, to remove it immediately, and to attack the invading infection with antibiotics, usually penicillin and streptomycin.

To identify the invading organism, culture samples are taken from the open sores, blood, urine, and sometimes the spinal fluid. Once the infection is under control, and the cause of the disease is removed, the white cell-producing tissues in the bone marrow recover and bring back a proper balance of white cells in the blood.

Agranulocytosis is also called *granulopenia, granulocytopenia, agranulytic angina, and malignant neutropenia. See also* LEUKOPENIA; WHITE BLOOD CELLS, DISEASES OF *and* **medigraph** LEUKEMIA.

**AGUE,** the name formerly used for *malaria.* Sometimes it is used loosely to describe any kind of shaking chills or spasm, and it may refer to neuralgic tics such as *tic douloureux. See also* NEURALGIA; TIC DOULOUREUX *and* **medigraph** MALARIA.